AF668116

HEALTHCARE COMMUNICATION AND SERVICES FOR MOTHER AND CHILD

HEALTHCARE COMMUNICATION AND SERVICES FOR MOTHER AND CHILD

Edited by

Dr. Satyajeet Nanda

KONARK PUBLISHERS PVT LTD
New Delhi • Seattle

Konark Publishers Pvt Ltd
206, First Floor, Peacock Lane,
Shahpur Jat,
New Delhi-110 049.
Phone: +91-11-41055065, 65254972
e-mail: india@konarkpublishers.com
Website: www.konarkpublishers.com

Konark Publishers International
1507 Western Avenue, #605,
Seattle, WA 98101
Phone: (415) 409-9988
e-mail: us@konarkpublishers.com

Copyright © Council for Social Development, New Delhi, 2011

All rights reserved. No part of this book may be reproduced or utilised in any form or by any means, electronic or mechanical, including photocopying, recording, or by any information storage and retrieval system, without prior permission in writing from the publishers.

Cataloging in Publication Data – DK
Courtesy: D.K. Agencies (P) Ltd. <docinfo@dkagencies.com>

Healthcare communication and services for mother and child / edited by Satyajeet Nanda.
p. cm.
Papers presented at a national seminar held at New Delhi in 2006.
Includes bibliographical references and index.
ISBN 8122007996

1. Maternal health services – India – Congresses. 2. Child health services – India – Congresses. 3. Medical policy – India – Congresses. 4. Communication in medicine – India – Congresses. 5. Medical personnel and patient – India – Congresses. I. Nanda, Satyajeet.

DDC 362.19820954 23

Editor: Seema Sreenivas
Typeset by The Laser Printers, New Delhi, and printed at ASK Advertising Aids Pvt Ltd, New Delhi.

Acknowledgements

At the outset let me express my gratitude to Prof. Muchkund Dubey and Dr N. J. Kurian of the Council for Social Development for supporting the concept of getting experts to a common discussion forum on very pertinent issues on healthcare. I also record my sincere thanks to Dr Pradipto Roy, Mr Sakarama, Dr Bhaswati, Dr Bimal Ch. Nanda and Mr Arun Ghosh for their support and suggestions at different phases.

My special thanks are due to the authors and reviewers of the papers. Specifically, thanks to Prof. Faujdar Ram (IIPS), Dr Sunita Reddy (JNU), Dr Satish Kumar Gupta (UNICEF), Dr Rajiv Dasgupta (JNU), Dr RR. Gangakhedkar (NARI), Dr Mohan Rao (JNU), Dr Sanghmitra Acharya (JNU), Dr T. R. Dilip (CDS), Shri Rattan Chand (MoHFW) and Dr Pradeep Panda for presenting studies on some of the most important facets of mother and child health. I am grateful to Prof P. M. Kulkarni, Ms Madhumita Das, Dr V. Jayachandran, Dr Gurumurthy Rangaiyan, Dr Debolina Mukherjee, Dr Anuradha De, Dr Hemant Meitei, Prof M. Vemuri, Mr B. K. Mishra and Mr K. B. Saxena for undertaking experts' review on the study findings and providing useful insights.

I record my thanks to the students of JNU, researchers at CSD, Madhumita Tripathy and Prof. A. K. Tripathy for giving their external suggestions on paper findings. I record my special thanks to Dr Mona K Jabbi, the current Director of CSD who plays a major role in publication of the book. I am also thankful to Mr R. S. Somi, Mr Rathor, Mr Bala and Mr Roy from CSD for their help in operational aspects of this publication.

Last, but not the least, thanks are due to the people behind the scene at different technical levels for their needful support.

February 5, 2011 **Satyajeet Nanda**

Contents

SECTION III
Specific Approaches towards Mother and Child Health

SECTION IV
Institutional Framework of Health Service: Issues of Power, Responsibility and Accountability

Contributors

Acharya, Sanghmitra S, Centre of Social Medicine and Community Health, School of Social Sciences, Jawaharlal Nehru University, New Delhi. E-mail: sanghmitraa@hotmail.com

Babille, Marzio, UNICEF, India Country Office, 73 Lodi Estate, New Delhi-110003.

Chand, Rattan, Department of Health and Family Welfare, Government of India, Nirman Bhavan, New Delhi. E-mail: pndt@nic.in

Dasgupta, Rajib, Centre of Social Medicine and Community Health, Jawaharlal Nehru University, New Delhi. E-mail: rdasgupta @mail.jnu.ac.in, dasgupta_jnu@yahoo.com

Dilip T. R., Centre for Development Studies, Prasanth Nagar Road, Ulloor, Thiruvananthapuram-695011, Telephone: 91-471-2448881-4, Fax: 91-471-2447137 E-mail: dilip@cds.ac.in

Gangakhedkar R. R: National AIDS Research Institute 73, G-Block, MIDC, Bhosari, Pune-411 026. E-mail: rgangakhedkar@nariindia.org

Gupta, Satish Kumar: UNICEF, India Country Office, 73 Lodi Estate, New Delhi.

Panda, Pradeep: Independent Consultant, New Delhi.

Nanda S: Social and Developmental Communications Unit, Mudra Inst. of Communication Research (MICORE), MICA, Shela village, Ahmedabad-380 058, India. E-mail: nsatyajeet@gmail.com; M: 09723120188

Nanda B: Consultant in Development Sector, Patamundai, Cuttack. E-mail: bnanda@sify.com

Rao, Mohan: Centre of Social Medicine and Community Health, JNU, New Delhi. E-mail: mohanrao@mail.jnu.ac.in

Reddy, Sunita: Centre of Social Medicine and Community Health, JNU, New Delhi. E-mail: sunitareddy@mail.jnu.ac.in

Tripathy-Nanda, Madhumita: Former Academic Associate (Nirma Univ.) Res. D-4 Sagun Jyoti, B/H. Dhanjay Tower, Satellite, Ahmedabad-15. E-mail: mmsntripathy@gmail.com

Introduction

One of the most important needs and hence indicator of development of human society is the health status of its constituents and mothers and children, in particular. In comparison to developed nations, South Asian countries, with their unique socio-political and economic structures, bear the responsibility of poorer situations in this regard. This is particularly so when there is a resource crunch or when the service is not easily available due to distance of the service-providing centres, unavailability of well-equipped/trained service providers or other reasons. Added to these factors are the cross cultural communication aspects in the form of culture-induced hesitations like collective shyness of women to visit male doctors in case of any gynaecological health problems. Similarly, children's healthcare also has its own unique problems.

A look into the past presents some of the hard facts on healthcare communication and service strategies of India. After Independence, the healthcare system particularly that of the mother and the child has been given much importance. This was done not only with regard to the extension of services but also in the very design of the healthcare system. Through various subsequent committees such as the Bhore Committee, Mudaliar Committee, Jain Committee, Kartar Singh Committee, Srivastava Committee to the recent NRHM model, India has strived to improve its health programmes.

The current scenario of mother and child health in India is somewhat disappointing, although some positive changes have taken place after colonial rule. With the introduction of various reform processes in different sectors of service delivery and creation of awareness, conditions have improved in some parts of the country. It is particularly visible in the southern states of India. But there are glaring disparities across regions and states. Many northern, central, and eastern states of India have continued to lag behind their southern counterparts in mother and child health status over decades. For example, infant-child mortality and morbidity and maternal mortality-morbidity situation have been extremely grave in states like Orissa, Madhya Pradesh, Assam etc. for the last three to four decades and they lag a great deal behind Kerala, Tamil Nadu etc. and even the country average. Orissa has been witnessing an infant mortality rate of more than 100 for more than three decades until a slight decline recently (83 as per 2005 SRS).

While different health system development programmes (HSDP) have upgraded different communication infrastructure, it has not helped people for optimal utilization of services. Health communicators have existed for quite some time in Indian health programmes for the last 60 years in different forms/names, such as *Gram Swasthya Mitra, Gram Swasthya Rakshak* and village health committee etc. The research question is, what works and in which circumstances i.e., credibility/applicability of the communication medium and differential in decision-making in different intervention programmes. It is observed that medicines from doctors and hospitals are not utilized due to lack of awareness/communication, in spite of the fact that health programmes have been supported by communication infrastructure and people response to health communication. In addition to it, lack of communication exists more at the grassroot level and this lead to underutilization of services. Government policy has not reached the people to an optimal extent due to problems in communication.

The backdrop of all these above facts finds a conglomeration of issues shrouding the healthcare communication and service system in India, particularly those catering to the needs of mother and child. There was, hence, a need felt for a brainstorming session which would facilitate debate, discussion, and mutual exchange of ideas and experiences among scholars and practitioners for diagnosing the issues and concerns afflicting the healthcare communication and service systems for the mother and the child. Such in-depth and systematic examination of the bottlenecks in policy and practice would, no doubt, lead to better prescriptions for eradicating the maladies afflicting the healthcare system and provide scope for improvements in areas where we have already achieved results.

It is in this context that the Council for Social Development held a National Seminar in 2006 at the India International Centre in New Delhi. A number of researchers from most states of India—north to south and east to west—contributed to a number of issues around healthcare service and communication. The seminar covered issues from maternal and child healthcare communication and utilization, disparities across regions and social categories, health finance, technologies, PPP and HIV/AIDS in India.

The scope of this book covers a broad perspective of mother and child health in India. In a disaggregated level the papers present four major sections:

SECTION I: Healthcare Service and Communication
SECTION II: Financing of Healthcare Services
SECTION III: Specific Approaches towards Mother and Child Health
SECTION IV: Institutional Framework of Health Service: Issues of Power, Responsibility and Accountability

In the first section of the book, the introductory paper by Nanda et al. on **'Mother and Child Health in India: Communication and Service Perspectives'** and the short documentary film (visual) on the gap between health service delivery and utilization in Orissa shows a grim picture of public health service both at systemic as well as individual levels. The paper sensitizes us about the importance of health communication and services and touches upon various theories such as Elaboration Likelihood Model, Health Belief Model, Protection Motivation Theory, Social Cognitive Theory, Social Support, Theory of Planned Behaviour/Reasoned Action, Transactional Model of Stress and Coping to explain the processes. The paper then takes a journey into the historical perspective of the health system in India right from the Mudaliar and Bhore committees to the recent NRHM frameworks. This is followed by a situation analysis of the current scenario of India that gives a comparative picture of different states of the country and identifies the pertinent issues and concerns in mother and child health in India. Finally the paper presents a case study of health communication and service in Orissa and reminds us of the basic concept of democracy that it is of the people, by the people and for the people.

In the same section of the book, Satish and Marzio in their paper **'Immunization Programmes for Mothers and Children:**

Achievements and Future Programmes', presented UNICEF's agenda of universal immunization. This paper has identified that both at the global level as well as in India a significant proportion of deaths among children, less than five years of age, occurs due to vaccine preventable diseases such as measles, neonatal tetanus, whooping cough etc... In case of women, tetanus toxoid (TT) injections can prevent deaths from neonatal tetanus. In spite of the fact that immunization is one of the most cost-effective public health interventions, a large proportion of vulnerable infants and children in India do not receive this simple intervention. In addition to an analysis of this situation, this paper also discusses the issues and challenges for the Millennium Development Goals and immunization coverage in India. It has posed some pertinent questions as to why India has not been able to achieve higher immunization coverage rates. The paper elaborates about the Multi-Year Plan for UIP, 2004-2009 by UNICEF, its vision, mission and specific strategies to achieve its goal.

Dasgupta rather tends to defend the concept of overdependence on UIP in his paper **'Vaccination Programmes: Limitations as a Universal Solution'** and adds issues behind the lagging vaccination programmes in India. He critically analyzes McKeown's argument on medical and heterogenous factors and spontaneous decline of infant mortality. In addition, the paper makes a situational analysis of the case of the Hepatitis B vaccine and oral polio vaccine programme of the Indian health system. The paper emphasizes on the limited role of vaccines in control of diseases and suggests an articulation of total package of the measures. Dasgupta sees immunization as "being oversold" ignoring the epidemiological complexities of diseases and cautions about the so called 'universal' solution rather than considering the realistic expectations in terms of its cost and human resource intensive operations.

In the second section of the book, Sanghmitra in her paper **'Financing Health-Some Issues and Concerns for Mother and Child'** presents the economics of healthcare system through different times and discusses about the health sector planning and mother and child health in terms of different frameworks such as MCH, CSSM, RCH and NRHM. The paper tries to locate the mother and child health programme in India's continuing Five-Year Plans and elaborates the health situation, service provisioning, sources of health finance and health expenditure. Sanghmitra aptly infers that although "... increasing public funding appears to be a better alternative to user fees... it is imperative to ensure quality care to the seekers/users."

Again in the second section of the book, Dilip in his paper **'Changing Patterns in Public Expenditure on Reproductive and Child Health Services in India'** discusses the public finance allocation and expenditure in health infrastructure and programme. It attempts to analyse the demand and supply components of public finance on health both at central and state government levels. The paper meticulously presents the source of funds for central and state government expenditure on RCH services and their utilization, and infers that components like urban family welfare services, training and research and evaluation require more attention and intensive analysis is necessary at regular intervals to ascertain the capacity of financing strategies in filling the gaps in access to RCH services across India.

In the third section of the book which focus on specific approaches in mother and child health, Sunita Reddy presents her paper on **'Health of Tribal Women and Children: A Holistic and Interdisciplinary Approach'**. This elaborates the health status of tribal women and children with specific focus on Tribes of Andaman and Nicobar Islands and critically analyses the use of inter-disciplinary approach to meet the challenges. She concludes that, "Stringent and strict laws should be made and implemented to protect the rights of the tribal people and policy related to use of forest lands, and health of the tribes should be favourable to the tribes."

In the same third section of the book, Gangakhedkar discusses a very important issue in his paper **'Mothers and Children affected by HIV/AIDS in India: Issues and Concerns'.** Giving us background information about the clinical components of HIV and the magnitude, the paper elaborates the natural history of HIV infection among women and Prevention of Mother to Child Transmission (PMTCT). Then the paper discusses the management of HIV disease in terms of use of ART, behaviour and drug adherence, social discrimination and coping up behaviour. With regard to programmatic response the paper infers that mothers and children affected by HIV pose a major challenge for the health system and the prevention of mother to child transmission strategies based on simple feasible single dose nevirapine are likely to limit maternal and paediatric therapeutic options.

In the fourth and final section of this book, Mohan Rao presents a critical analysis of policies in his paper **'A Red Herring: Population Policies and Maternal Health in Neo-Liberal Times'.** This paper strongly criticizes the loopholes in the government systems at policy level and infers that the initiatives may lead to the decline of the state, the rise in fundamentalism and anti-feminism and the focus on population then serves as a red herring.

In the same section, Pradeep Panda examines the role of Panchayati Raj institutions in decentralized governance and healthcare with a specific case study of Kerala's health sector under decentralization. Rattan Chand in his paper **'Pre-conception and Pre-natal Diagnostic Techniques Act 1994 – Its Need, Features and Implementation Status'** presents the government standpoints on the practical aspects of how at implementation level the Pre-conception and Pre-natal Diagnostic Techniques Act 1994 has been used in India.

Since the book provides a broader picture of the concepts, components and perspectives of mother and child health in India, it will be useful for a large number of readers and stakeholders. On the one hand, this will provide a conceptual framework for systems related academic studies while, on the other hand, this will impinge upon the researchers to carry out further disaggregate investigations at the micro and macro level. Policy-makers, programme managers and community level workers can utilize the book to its utmost to design and implement interventions.

SECTION I

Healthcare Service and Communication

1

Mother and Child Health in India: Communication and Service Perspectives

S. Nanda, B. Nanda and Madhumita Tripathy-Nanda

1. Importance of Health Communication and Services

Healthcare is one of the prime sectors, which a modern welfare state can ill-afford to neglect. Particularly, the health of the mother and the child is very important as the child is a proto-citizen of a country and the mother is the root, which nurtures and nourishes this future citizen. Any aspiration towards the development of human resources of a nation-state is, hence, bound to end up as a pipe dream unless adequate healthcare services are provided to the mother and the child during appropriate periods of their life cycles.

When it comes to the countries of South Asia, certain peculiarities of the socio-political and economic structures make it almost an inevitable responsibility on the part of the state to take special care of the health of its women and children. India, for instance, is a country where the ideology of patriarchy is deep rooted not only in the sphere of culture but also in the arenas of decision-making (both in the private sphere of home and the public sphere that lies beyond the home environment) and ownership/control of private property. In the family, it is the health, education and food/nutritional needs of the male adults, which are given ascendancy over the same needs of the females. This is particularly so when there is some kind of resource crunch or when the service is not easily available due to distance of the service-providing centres, unavailability of well-equipped/trained service providers or any other reasons. Added to these factors are the culture-induced hesitations like the collective shyness on the part of women to visit male doctors in case there is some reproductive health problem.

Health communication has developed over the last twenty-five years as a vibrant and important field of study concerned with the powerful roles performed by human and mediated communication in healthcare delivery and health promotion. Health communication inquiry has emerged as an exciting applied behavioural science research area. It is an applied area of research not only because it examines the pragmatic influences of human communication on the provision of healthcare and the promotion of public health, but also because the work in this area is often used to enhance the quality of healthcare delivery and health promotion. To this end, health communication inquiry is usually problem-based, focusing on identifying, examining, and solving healthcare and health promotion problems.

Within the health communication field, communication is conceptualized as the central social process in the provision of healthcare delivery and the promotion of public health. The centrality of the process of communication is based upon the pervasive roles communication performs in creating, gathering, and sharing 'health information.' Health information is the most important resource in healthcare and health promotion because it is essential in guiding strategic health behaviours, treatments, and decisions (Kreps, 1988).

Health communication in its literal form links the domains of communication and health and is increasingly recognized as a necessary element of efforts to improve personal and public health. Health communication can contribute to all aspects of disease prevention and health promotion, and is relevant in a number of contexts. There are various theories of health communication. They describe different contexts and components of the process in which different factors play roles and ultimately decide the nature of communication. Some of them are Elaboration Likelihood Model, Health Belief Model, Protection Motivation Theory, Social Cognitive Theory, Social Support, Theory of Planned Behaviour/Reasoned Action, Transactional Model of Stress and Coping etc.

The problem of children's healthcare has a certain typicality of its own but it has not yet cut off the umbilical cord that it shares with the mother's. In fact, the interventions made to improve mother's health during pregnancy, labour and delivery have had a positive impact on pregnancy outcome and child health (Pachauri, 1996:255).[1] Early childhood healthcare like immunization and proper supply of nutrition are also essential ingredients for development of the child into a healthy adult.

While discussing healthcare services for mother and child, one should not be oblivious of the fact that women or children as a whole are not homogeneous categories. There are gaps in the supply, demand and utilities of healthcare services among women and children of different socio-economic backgrounds, for instance, between the rich and poor, rural and urban, among different social groups like SCs/STs/Minorities and other population etc. Thus, the time has come to take another look at the healthcare services for mother and child from different perspectives.

2. Historical Perspective

After independence, the healthcare system particularly that of mother and child has been given much importance in India. This was done not only with regard to the extension of services but also in the design of the healthcare system. Way back in 1946, the Bhore Committee report spelt out the foundations of the healthcare system in India in terms of norms regarding infrastructure and personnel. In several respects, the Bhore Committee Report was similar to the Beveridge Committee report of UK which formed the basis for the celebrated National Health Service of that country. It clearly enunciated the population to be covered under block, taluka and district level hospitals/health centres, number of doctors, number of beds and nurses to be allotted to them etc. Major emphasis was on preventive measures with a pro-community approach. After the Bhore Committee, many other special committees were formed to cater to further healthcare needs of people and necessary modifications and additions were carried out.

The Mudaliar Committee in 1961 emphasized the strengthening of the PHC and more clearly designing its structure according to population size. This committee also stressed the central government's role in combating communicable diseases and establishment of medical colleges. Then came the Jain Committee in 1966 which put more emphasis on taluka level heath services and enhancing maternity facilities at all levels of the healthcare system. A major hallmark of this committee was that it took into consideration the issue of health insurance for the first time. In 1974, the Kartar Singh Committee report gave primacy to the PHC. To provide MCH services at PHC level, this committee recommended for an additional doctor at PHC level assisted by one or more nurses. Even at lower levels, one male and one female health worker were proposed for a population of 5000. In 1975, the Srivastava Committee recommended for the establishment of a medical and health education commission. This committee also put forth a proposal to increase the PHC level drug budget.

In 1980 a joint panel of ICMR and ICSSR focused on village healthcare services and recommended for village health workers from both sexes. Sub-centres were identified to be village level health centres covering 5,000 of the population. At the block level, CHCs were recommended for catering to the healthcare needs of 10,000 of the population, and six general doctors and three specialists were to be deputed to the CHC. One district health centre was to cover one million of the population and specialist centres were to cover a population of five million. In its proposal, this panel earmarked six per cent of the GNP to be spent on the healthcare services. The first National Health Policy of India was prepared in 1983. This exclusively designed the health infrastructure to streamline health services delivery at all levels. This also focused on training of health workers at village level. Health and demographic targets were specified and a decentralized health system was emphasized. Involvement of NGOs and private sector in health service delivery was recognized and encouraged.

One of the recent developments related to maternal and child healthcare service is the National Population Policy 2000. It has its clear stands on the demographic outcomes of reproductive and child healthcare in all parts of the country. More machinery has been developed for a decentralized structure of healthcare system. Panchayati raj institutions, the private sector, NGOs and other community groups have been considered to be partners in healthcare service deliveries for a better mother and child health situation. The most recent steps being the Rural Health Mission by the central government which focuses on mother and child healthcare in rural areas with community participation.

3. Current Scenario of India

The situation of mother and child health in India is quite disappointing, although some positive changes have taken place after independence. With the introduction of various reform processes in different sectors of service delivery and creation of awareness, the condition has improved in some parts of the country. It is particularly visible in the southern part of India. Still disparities across regions and states are quite clear. Many northern, central, and eastern states of India have lagged behind their southern counterparts in mother and child health status over decades. For example, infant-child mortality and morbidity and maternal mortality-morbidity situation have been extremely grave in states like Orissa, Madhya Pradesh, Assam etc... for the last three to four decades and they lag a great deal behind Kerala, Tamil Nadu etc... and even the country average. Orissa has been witnessing an infant mortality rate of more than 100 for more than three decades until a slight decline recently (83 as per 2005 SRS).[2] Likewise, fertility rates have been at very high levels in Uttar Pradesh, Madhya Pradesh, Bihar and Rajasthan, and much poorer than south Indian states. The said northern states have TFR (total fertility rate) of more than 3.0, whereas the southern states have already achieved fertility transition with fertility less than 2.2.

Many other aspects of maternal and child health also show a gloomy picture in different parts of the country. The magnitude of safe delivery, ANC and immunization coverage is quite lower in many states of India (NFHS, 1998-99). The prevalence of reproductive morbidity, infertility and unsafe abortion too show a high level of disparity in some parts of the country (NFHS, 1998-99). The sex ratio of India as well as some of the economically advanced states like Haryana, Punjab, Gujarat and Delhi has been found to be disadvantageous to females. Then, there is the case of advanced medical technology being misused/abused by some unscrupulous members of the medical fraternity to swell their coffers taking advantage of deep-rooted superstitions and social evils. A case in point is the Pre-natal Diagnostic Test being used to determine the sex of the foetus which often leads to female foeticide. In fact, this is one of the reasons cited for the dismal sex ratio in some of the north

Indian states. This is not withstanding the fact that the original objective of this test was to take stock of the situation in case there were some congenital disorders found in the foetus.

Thus we find a conglomeration of issues shrouding the healthcare service system in India, particularly those catering to the needs of the mother and the child. There is, hence, a need for a brain-storming which would facilitate debate, discussion, and mutual exchange of ideas and experiences among scholars and practitioners for diagnosing the issues and concerns afflicting the healthcare service systems for the mother and the child. Such in-depth and systematic examination of the bottlenecks in policy and practice would, no doubt, lead to better prescriptions for eradicating the maladies afflicting the healthcare system and provide scope for improvements in areas where we have already achieved. It is in this context that the Council for Social Development conducted a National Seminar on issues and concerns in Mother and Child healthcare services in India.

4. Pertinent Issues and Concerns in Indian Context

In the last few decades, a number of research works has been carried out across the length and breadth of issues of healthcare service and communication that address the following major ones:

a. Supply, access, quality, affordability, delivery and utilization of services.
b. Disparities in services among different regions and social categories like SCs/STs/minorities etc.
c. Financing of healthcare services for mother and child: Taking stock of the present and projecting into the future.
d. Immunization programmes for children: Problems and prospects.
e. New technologies for maternal and child health services like pre-natal diagnostics tests: Issues of use and abuse.
f. Role of Panchayati Raj institutions: Issues of power and privilege, responsibility and accountability.
g. Privatization of services: Dilemma facing a welfare state.
h. Mothers and children affected by HIV/AIDS in India: Issues and concerns.

5. A Case Study of Health Communication and Service in Orissa

The maternal and child health conditions in Orissa have continued to be grave over the decades. The maternal and child mortality rates in Orissa have been at much higher magnitude than the national averages and their infant mortality rate (IMR) is the highest among all the states of India (IMR was 83 in the year 2003).[3] A study (Nanda *et al.* 1999) has shown that many of the supply (financial constraint, geo-physical disadvantages) and demand (poor awareness level) factors can significantly influence the utilization of available health services.

At a conceptual level, Kennedy's adaptive behaviour model and Rossenstock's health belief model converge with the researcher's viewpoint. Kennedy suggests that within any workable environment, human beings display different kinds of behaviour that provide a workable adaptation to the threat of a disease and other health-related problems. Similarly, Rossenstock is of the view that a person feels motivated to go for preventive practices to avoid disease only if he/she believes that he/she is susceptible to the disease and that the occurrence of the disease would have severe repercussions on him/her.[4] It implies that availability of health services in the neighbourhood may act as one of the prime factors which influence the individual families' approach towards seeking/utilizing RCH services. Thus there is the possibility of the existence of a linkage among the trinity of *supply, demand and utility vis-à-vis health communication* of RCH services due to the presence of certain intervening factors. Against these backdrops the current study aims to study the level of maternal and child health service utilization and problems faced by the people in public and private sector health systems.

Taking into consideration the level of maternal and child health conditions, Sambalpur, a major district of Orissa, was selected for study. The district is divided into nine blocks. On the basis of the available health system and infrastructure, maternal and child health condition and remoteness from urban area, two blocks nearer to and two blocks far from the district headquarter were chosen for study. So out of the nine blocks, four blocks viz...Dhankauda, Maneswar, Jujomura and Rengali were selected. Then from these selected blocks some villages (PSUs) were identified following PPS (probability proportion to size) sampling method. So, 10 villages were selected. On an average 25 households (SSUs) were identified for interview from each selected village through Systematic Random Sampling method. So a total of 250 households covering a population of 1337 were interviewed. A well-designed, pre-coded and pre-tested structured questionnaire was used for interviews in the survey. In addition to the sample survey, some qualitative methods, such as focus group discussions (FGD), non-participant observation, in-depth interviews were utilized to collect necessary information from community members and key-informants to supplement the data. The data collection was carried out during 2005-2006.

Socio-economic, Demographic and Ethnographic Profile of Study Population

In Sambalpur district the proportion of Scheduled Caste population to the total is 17.04 per cent and that of the Scheduled Tribe population is 34.5 per cent. There are around 64 types of Scheduled Castes and 50 types of Scheduled Tribes in the district. Among the Scheduled Tribes, Kisans, Orams, Mirdhas, Hos, Mundas and Kharias, Gonds, Kandha, Binjhal, Kudas are the major ones. Among the Scheduled Castes, Pano and Hadi caste constituted the major proportion and others being the Dhoba, Kela, Keuta and Domb. Unlike other Scheduled Tribe groups in the sample Kondh, Munda and Kissan tribes seemed to be more or less the primordial aborigines of the district. The Scheduled Tribes have a kind of formal social structure with a set of societal folkways. The food habits, marital lifestyle, rituals in life-cycle events (puberty, marriage, childbirth and death) are often influenced by societal norms. Even sexual behaviour such as abstinence, frequency etc... are also affected by cultural values. In contrast, the Schedules Castes at present don't have such a rigid formal social structure with rigid societal norms followed. Marriage and sharing of lifestyle outside one's own caste are also common in Scheduled Castes.

It was found that around 49 per cent of the total population is in the reproductive age group i.e., 15-49 years, while more than 40 per cent of the total population is below 15 years of age. Little less than 12 per cent of all have crossed the age of 50. The following table shows that 40 per cent of the total sample population is dependent upon the rest of the people who are the earning members. Of the

Table 1: Socio-economic Profile (N=1337)

Variables	Per cent
Age in yrs.	
0	5.8
1-5	19.6
6-14	14.1
15-49	48.8
50 +	11.7
Sex	
Male	51.9
Female	48.1
Marital status	
Unmarried	47.6
Currently married	48.4
Divorced/separated	0.1
Widowed/widower	3.8
Education	
Illiterate	45.0
Class 1-5	21.8
Class 6-10	19.1
Class 11-12	4.6
Graduate	1.6
Post-Graduate or higher degree	0.4
Technical qualification/other professional degrees/diplomas	0.4
literate but no formal education	7.0
Occupation	
Agriculture	5.7
Service	3.9
Business/self-employed	9.4
Wage labour	17.7
Others	63.3
Caste/tribe	
ST	47.6
SC	30.4
OBC	16.4
Others	5.2

total more than 25 per cent are children below the age of six. The sex ratio of the sample population is slightly tilted in favour of the males. The proportion of males is 52 per cent while for females it is 48 per cent. The difference between the proportion of currently married and unmarried persons is very small as it is less than 1 per cent. The proportion of currently married persons is slightly less than the 50 per cent mark.

About 45 per cent of the total population is illiterate. Only two per cent of the total population is either a graduate or a post-graduate. Less than 0.5 per cent of the population has any technical qualification/other professional degrees/diplomas. Dropouts seem to be high as it was found that the number of students decreased with each higher class. A very remarkable feature is that seven per cent of the population is literate without any formal education, meaning, AWWs and some other agencies might be playing some role in providing education. The occupational structure of the sample population shows that 18 per cent of them are wage labourers, followed by ten per cent in business/self-employed people. A huge percentage (63.3 per cent) is in 'others' category which means their occupation is very tentative or they are simply not earning which includes students, housewives etc. Low level of education is also reflected in the fact that the percentage of the population engaged in services is below four. Similarly the percentage of people engaged in agriculture falls below six as most of them do not have a piece of land to cultivate. Maximum number of households belongs to Scheduled Tribes who comprise more than 47 per cent of the total household respondents. More than 30 per cent of the respondents are from the Scheduled Castes, while 16.4 per cent belonged to the Other Backward Classes. Only 5.2 per cent of the total households interviewed are from general caste.

Table 2: Proportion of Health Expenditure to Total Annual Expenditure

Per cent of total expenditure	Frequency	Per cent of households
0-15	168	67.2
15.1-25	49	19.6
25.1-40	16	6.4
40.1 +	17	6.8
Total	250	100

Figure 1 shows the proportion of total expenditure, sample households spend towards their health only. A majority of them spend within 15 per cent, whereas around one-fifth of all sample households spend between 15-25 per cent of their total annual

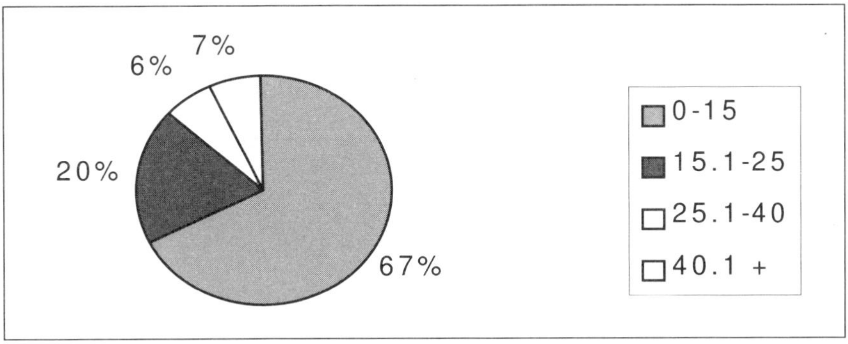

Figure 1: Proportion of Health Expenditure

expenditure towards health. Even around seven per cent of all reported to have spent as high as 40 per cent or more in this respect.

Table 3: Demographic Profile of Sample Households (N=250)

Variables	Per cent
Currently married women in 15-45 years	
0	5.2
1	80.0
2 +	14.8
Pregnant women in the HH	
0	90.0
1	10.0
Children 0-5 yrs	
0	16.4
1	49.6
2	24.4
3 +	9.6
Child delivery/abortion in last 2 yrs	
0	41.2
1	50.0
2	7.2
3	1.6

It was found that more than 80 per cent of all households have only one currently married woman in the 15-45 years age group. Even 15 per cent of all households have two or more such women. It was found that in more than five per cent of the households there is not a single currently married woman in 15-45 years age group. It was found that ten per cent of the sample households have one or more pregnant woman. Around half of all households have children who are a year old, while 25 per cent have children of two or more years of age. Little more than 16 per cent of all households have infant children. Again in half of all sample households there has been one child delivery/abortion in the last two years. In more than 40 per cent of the cases there has been no pregnancy/abortion in the last two years. Around nine per cent of the households had two delivery/abortions in the last two years, which reflect a higher fertility rate for these households.

Health Status of Mother and Child

As already described in the beginning, health of mother and child is an essential aspect of development and is dependent on many factors. Some of the important ones are quality and quantity of service delivery and their proper utilization. We will now discuss the maternal and child health services utilization by community in a rural set-up. To know the utilization fully, one needs to start with the kind of illness to mother and child or their health status, treatment seeking, information given to people about services and illness, quality of available healthcare service and more importantly people's perceptions, their problems and reported suggestions. All these aspects have been studied keeping a short reference period of one year to avoid the problem of recall lapse.

Table 4: Prevalence of Illness and Treatment Seeking (N=250)

Variables	Per cent
Frequency of illness to women/ children during last 1 year	
1-3 times	30.0
4-7 times	38.8
More than 7 times	26.4
Never	4.8
Prevalence of illness*	
Fever	45.6
Diarrhoea/Dysentery/Loose Motion	41.2
Malaria	25.2
Cold/cough	45.6
Anaemia/Weakness	6.4
Back pain during pregnancy/in general	12.8

(Contd.)

Variables	Per cent
Gastric problem	1.6
Itching	5.6
Menstruation	4.4
Brain Malaria	1.2
Measles	2.8
Jaundice	4.4
Vomiting	.4
TB	.8
Gyneac/Obstet problems	4.4
Other	12.4
Woman and child reported to have Illness*	
Woman	81.2
Child	65.6
Frequency of medicine/treatment taken by women/children last 2yrs	
1-3 times	48.4
4-7 times	28.4
More than 7 times	18.4
Never	4.8
Source of treatment*	
No treatment	28.8
Allopath	89.6
Ayurvedic	1.2
Other professionals	0.4
Hakim	3.6
Self-treatment	1.2
Other	0.4
Reasons for not seeking treatment*	
No knowledge of service	2.8
Not necessary	7.2
Financial constraint	14.0
No support structure to go out	2.8
Other reasons	1.6

*means percentages do not add to 100 due to multiple answers.

Regarding the frequency of illness to women/children of the sample households during the last one year it was found that in as high as 38.8 per cent of the sample households, women/children fall sick four to seven times, while only five per cent of them said that no women/children had fallen ill in the last one year. In more than 26 per cent of the households, women/children fell ill more than seven times in the last one year. Among the diseases, the highest proportion (45 per cent) reported to have had fever. Diarrhoea/ dysentery/loose motions are the second most frequently occurring diseases reported by 41 per cent of the total affected ones. This may be the reason why diarrhoea has been identified as one of main causes of child deaths in Orissa. Cold/cough is found to be very common in the areas under survey. More than one-fourth of the patients are infected by deadly malaria. Even back pain, menstrual and gynaecological problems have been report by some people.

It is found that more than 90 per cent of the people give spontaneous answers regarding their diseases, while 23 per cent of the people answer on probing reflecting a lower level of awareness/ concern about their own health problems. Around 81.2 per cent women reported to have been affected by different illness/disease than the children. However, as high as 65 per cent of all children are affected by various diseases.

Treatment Seeking Behaviour

It is important to know about the treatment seeking behaviour in order to understand the health service utilization. Hence a study was undertaken on the sources and frequency of treatment, reasons for not treating etc. in detail again keeping a short reference period of one year to avoid the problem of recall lapse. The findings are presented below.

It was found that only 18.8 per cent of the households sought any medicine for affected women/children more than seven times compared to more than 26 per cent of them who fall ill these many times (as shown previously in the first table). It means a large number of people are not going for treatment even though they are ill. Only five per cent of the respondents have reported not to have ever sought any medicine/treatment for their women/children. About 90 per cent go for treatments from allopathic doctors, while only 1.2 per cent prefers ayurvedic doctors. An important finding is that nearly 29 per cent of them go without any treatment. Financial constraints have obstructed majority (14 per cent) of the patients from taking any treatment. However, 7.2 per cent did not feel the necessity of taking any treatment and no knowledge of service has been the reason for three per cent of them for not seeking any treatment.

Health Information and Communication

It is very important to impart correct, clear and precise information about illness, treatment and available health services so as to get a healthy population. This is an area which has grossly been undermined in many parts of India and consequently we have visibly poor utilization of services added with poor health status. These aspects have been studied taking a short reference period of two years to avoid possible recall lapse. Around 82 per cent of the sample households have received some kind of information regarding mother and child health services. That means close to one-fifth of the whole population has absolutely not been given any information on health services available. So the repercussions have to be grave.

Among them who received health information, little more than half reported to have got it from the anganwadi workers (AWWs). While 23.2 per cent of the respondents receive information from people, around 19 per cent are benefited from village health workers/ ANM in this respect. Around 14 per cent of the sample households get information from the government doctors. The media plays little role and NGOs have almost no contribution in providing health information to people. It is found that ANC and immunization are comparatively known more to the people, although as low as 47 per cent and 42 per cent respectively, when government continues to see its goal for 100 per cent coverage. Only 18 per cent have received any information about family planning and only 10 per cent about safe delivery. It seems information on treatment of infertility, abortion, and treatment of reproductive morbidity is not provided to people as reflected from the reporting as below two per cent.

Table 5: Health Information to Sample Households (N=250)

Variables	Per cent
Information given on mother and child health services in last 2 yrs	82.4
Sources of health information*	
TBA	1.6
Village health worker/ANM	18.8
Media	12.8
Govt. doctor	14.4
Private doctor	9.2
People	23.2
NGO	1.6
AWW	50.8

(Contd.)

Variables	Per cent
Kind of information received*	
Family planning	18.0
ANC (TT, IFA, BP, Weight, Nutrition)	47.2
Safe delivery	10.4
PNC (breast-feeding, nutrition, infant and women's healthcare)	5.6
Immunization	42.0
Treatment of infertility	1.6
Abortion	1.6
Treatment of reproductive morbidity, STI/STD	1.6
Others	8.4
People heard about health service/schemes available in the district*	
Girl child benefit	26.0
ORS	62.4
Family planning	5.2
ANC	18.0
PNC	2.4
Weekly Immunization	24.8
Hepatitis-B	3.6
Jaundice	1.6
Menstrual problem	1.2
STI/STD/HIV-AIDS	0.4
Janani surakshya yojana	1.6
Source of information about health service/schemes in the district*	
Posters	2.0
Radio/TV	17.6
People	39.0
TBA/ANM/Village health worker	2.0
Hospitals	16.6
Any other (specify)	22.9

*means percentage does not add to 100 due to multiple answers.

In this study, information on specific schemes/services launched or currently in function, related to mother and child health, was collected from hospitals and other district level official sources. When asked about the same schemes/services to the sample households, ORS seemed to be the most popular which is known to more than 62 per cent households. One-fourth of the households have heard about the weekly immunization programme. Little more than one-fourth of all study households knew about the 'Girl Child Benefit scheme' in which a mother gets some money after delivery of a girl child. However, this is almost not functional now. 39 per cent of households get information from people. Around 18 per cent of households get health information from the radio/TV, while 17 per cent get to know from the hospitals.

CASE STUDY 1

Informant's age:	28 years
Sex:	female
Occupation:	basket making
Caste:	ST
Village:	Mundher

Kuntala, the respondent, was married when she was eight years old in the year 1998. She has delivered four children out of which only one survives till now and the rest have died during infancy. She delivered her first infant son in April 1999. The baby survived for two days only. Immediately after birth the baby suffered from high fever and skin rashes. The child delivery had taken place at home and there was no doctor in the village or nearby to treat him. Nobody in the whole village could diagnose the illness, not even the traditional healer. The respondent and her husband being poor basket-makers could not afford to go to doctors in town. Financial constraints, lack of transport facility and no medical treatment subsequently led to the tragic death of the two-day-old infant son.

This was not the last incident for Kuntala. She had to face a similar trauma of losing another baby daughter. That baby daughter was born to her one year after the death of her first infant son. This time the new-born daughter died even earlier, i.e., within 24 hours after birth. Kuntala was very weak and anaemic during her second pregnancy. The infant daughter was light weight and anaemic too. This delivery too had taken place at home, and "....probably that is the reason why the infant daughter died within 24 hours without getting any medical supervision...".

The third child of Kuntala is still surviving and is now a four-year-old boy. But the fourth one born after this is another sad story. In June 2005 she had delivered another baby boy who died of jaundice seven days after birth.

Three infant mortalities !! From one family !!! Poor Kuntala had to face all these tragic incidents due to lack of medical and transport facilities.

CASE STUDY 2

Name of the Informant:	Pramila Bag
Occupation:	Housewife
Age:	30 years
Village:	Golabandh
Caste:	Keuta

Mrs Pramila Bag is a resident of the village Golabandh which comes under the Maneswar block of Sambalpur district of Orissa. She is a victim of the deadly disease cancer i.e., ovarian cancer. She has two children, one boy, who is eight years of age and another girl child who is four years of age. According to her version, both deliveries were normal and took place at home in the village under the medical supervision of the ANM of Golabandh. Pramila says, after one year of her second delivery, she suddenly started getting pain in her lower abdomen. In course of time the pain became intolerable and she went to Sambalpur. But as she was poor and uneducated the doctors recommended some medicines without performing any medical tests. She brought some medicines and took them for ten days and then stopped as the medicines were very expensive. Her lower abdominal pain persisted. Pramila was advised by the ANM to seek treatment in Burla Medical Hospital. Pramila went to Burla and she was advised to do some medical tests by the gynaecologist. After the medical tests it was confirmed that she suffered from ovarian cancer. She is still surviving but has no money for further treatment of this disease. There is no doctor in her village and the medicines prescribed to her are costly. Nobody knows how long she is going to survive.

6. Summary and Implications

With the alarmingly high rate of maternal and child mortality and morbidity vis-à-vis poorer level of overall performance of Orissa state in health sector, it was felt important to carry out an exploratory study on service delivery and utilisation. It was aimed to study the health governance including the programmes and service delivery, on the one hand, and the service utilisation by the community, on the other. The Sambalpur district of Orissa state was taken as a case study, in which the samples were drawn from 250 households from ten villages situated in four blocks. Information was collected from both community and health staffs.

Analyses showed that majority of the people that is little less than half of all belong to the reproductive age group of 15-49 years and one-fourth are infant and child population. The sex ratio is a little disadvantageous towards females. Little less than half are currently married. On education, 45 per cent of the total is illiterate and do not know how to read and write. That is the reason why the percentage of the population engaged in services is below four. Similarly, the percentage of people engaged in agriculture falls below six as most of them do not have a piece of land to cultivate or are small land-holders. Primary occupation of most people is wage labour.

The disadvantageous situation with regard to house type, kitchen, place for livestocks, sewage disposal and drinking water have been substantiated with the reported findings of diarrhoea and skin infections. The health service providers are mostly between 37–59 years of age, working for the last 10–20 years. On health status, in as high as 38.8 per cent of the sample households, women/children fall sick four to seven times. Close examination of people's actual reporting of illness and treatment behaviour reveals that many people seem to be less aware in perceiving their illness and also about treatment. Malaria and diarrhoea are the most frequently occurring diseases reported by households. This may be the fact that diarrhoea has been identified as one of the main causes of many of the child deaths occurring in Orissa. Patients suffered for more than ten days. It reflects the quality of treatment and immunity level available with the affected mother and children. Large numbers of people are not going for treatment even though they are ill. Nearly 29 per cent of them go without any treatment. Financial constraints have obstructed a majority (14 per cent) of the patients from taking any treatment.

It is shocking to find that more than 17 per cent of the population has absolutely not received any communication about existence of health services around them. Half of all respondents say that they receive health information from the *anganwadi* workers. The media has lesser contribution and NGOs have almost no contribution in providing health information. In terms of health information, only ten per cent got information about safe delivery, being one of the most important aspects of mother and child healthcare. ORS seems to be the most and, maybe, the only popular health service available. Most people seek health services from private allopath clinics. Although government plans to strengthen the SC and PHC, the services are extremely less utilized from them even by villagers. The coverage of TT, IFA, institutional delivery and child immunization etc. warns us that we are still far from our government's goal of 100 per cent coverage. Long distances to health facilities, lack of proper transport facilities and severe financial constraints are responsible for these.

These findings are very important for programme managers while taking care of health planning. In these contexts new developments like ASHA training, specific programmes for specific groups are reported to be innovations. This not only reminds us but also questions the very concept of democracy as "of the people, by the people and for the people."

NOTES

1. Pachauri. S, 'A Shift from Family Planning to Reproductive Health: New Challenges' in Srinivasan, K. (ed.) *Population Policy and Reproductive Health*, Hindustan Publishing Corporation, New Delhi, 1996.
2. Registrar-General of India (2005): *SRS Bulletin*, Sample Registration System, 39 (1)
3. SRS Bulletin, April 2005.
4. For further understanding, see S.R.Mehta, 1987.

REFERENCES

1. Government of India, Census of India: Provisional Population Totals, Series 22: Orissa Paper 2, Directorate of Census Operations, Orissa, 2001.
2. International Institute for Population Sciences and ORC Macro, National Family Health Survey (NFHS-2), 1998-99, IIPS, Mumbai, 2000.
3. International Institute for Population Sciences, RHS-Reproductive and Child Health, Orissa 1998-99, IIPS, Mumbai, 2002.
4. Local Public Health Governance Performance Assessment Instrument (2006): http://www.cdc.gov/od/ocphp/nphpsp/Documents/Governance Evaluation.pdf (visited on 12th May 2006).
5. Mehta S. R., Society and Health: A Sociological Perspective, Rawat Publication, 1987.
6. Nanda S. et.al, 'Utilization of Antenatal Care (ANC) Service by the Scheduled Tribes in India', *Journal of Human Ecology*, 10 (2): 99-104, 1999.
7. Orissa Human Development Report, Some Measures of Human Development: An Inter-district Analysis, Directorate of Economic and Statistics, Orissa, 2004.

8. Pandey Arvind, Minja Kim Choe, Norman Y. Luther, D. Sahu and Jagdish Chand, 'Infant and Child Mortality in India', National Family Health Survey Subject Reports No. 11, International Institute for Population Sciences, Mumbai, India and East-West Center Program on Population, Honolulu, Hawaii, USA, 1998.
9. Patil A.V. et.al, 'Current Health Scenario in Rural India', *Australian Journal of Rural Health*, 10(2), 129-135, 2002.
10. 'Programming Reproduction? Maternal health services' (2005): www.hsph.harvard.edu/organisation/healthnet/SAsia/suchana/0804/rh347.html (visited on 27 July 2005).
11. Registrar-General of India, *SRS Bulletin*, Sample Registration System, 39 (1), 2005
12. Sanghvi T. G, 'Reaching Every Child Now', *Global Health Link*, May-June, p.12, 2004.

2

Immunization Programmes for Mothers and Children: Achievements and Future Programmes

Dr. Satish Kumar Gupta and Dr. Marzio Babille

Executive Summary

Immunization and vaccines have brought innovation and science to children and women in all countries and represent one of the most successful and cost-effective public health stories in history. Immunization has wiped out smallpox, substantially reduced morbidity and mortality from diphtheria, pertussis, tetanus and measles, and is on the verge of eradicating polio. Since its inception in 1974, the Expanded Programme on Immunizations (EPI) has provided guidance and recommendations to national authorities on how to design, develop and manage immunization services to efficiently deliver needed immunizations. Thanks to the establishment of strong immunization services, over two-thirds of the world's targeted population is now reached with immunizations.

Of global deaths among children, less than five years of age, a significant proportion dies of vaccine preventable diseases. These include 770,000 deaths due to measles and 200,000 deaths due to neonatal tetanus.[1] Many of these children are already otherwise compromised by malnutrition or other infectious diseases. In a country like India, by vaccinating 1000 infants we can prevent around 30 deaths from measles and ten deaths from whooping cough.

Vaccinating 1000 women with tetanus toxoid (TT) prevents five deaths from neonatal tetanus. Immunization is one of the most cost-effective public health interventions available. Yet, a large proportion of vulnerable infants and children in India are not receiving this simple intervention. Across India in 2001-02, only 63.6 per cent of children between 12-23 months had received all six of their primary vaccines, with a wide variation among states.[2] States with poorer immunization rates generally have higher child mortality rates. India has also the largest number of infants who reach their first birthday not fully immunized. (Estimated at nearly 18 million for the 2001 birth cohort). Surveillance quality tends to be worst in areas with lowest coverage. So, reported diseases represent only a small fraction of actual disease incidence. Despite these problems, incidence of Universal Immunization Programme (UIP) diseases has substantially decreased since 1985. But, much work remains to protect all of India's children from these preventable diseases. The size and diversity of India make this especially challenging as do resource constraints and competing priorities.

Achieving high immunization coverage and sustaining it is one of the main challenges for the Millennium Development Goals (MDGs) when coverage data indicates that performance is slipping back. The frontline strategy should be to reach the unreached and accelerate disease control efforts—polio eradication, NNT elimination and measles control.

The effectiveness of immunization is thoroughly proven. Unlike most other health and development interventions, immunization does not simply raise the chances that children will resist a disease: it virtually guarantees they will. Each year since 1990, routine immunization with vaccine against diphtheria, pertussis and tetanus has reached more than 70 per cent of all children, an extraordinary accomplishment considering that more than 130 million children are born each year and need to be immunized. Combined with accelerated disease control programmes, routine services have contributed significantly to child survival, averting more than two million deaths a year and preventing countless episodes of illness and disability.

Introduction

Immunization and vaccines have brought innovation and science to children and women in all countries and represent one of the most successful and cost-effective public health stories in history. Immunization has wiped out smallpox, substantially reduced morbidity and mortality from diphtheria, pertussis, tetanus and measles, and is on the verge of eradicating polio. Since its inception in 1974, the Expanded Programme on Immunizations (EPI) has provided guidance and recommendations to national authorities on how to design, develop, and manage immunization services to efficiently deliver needed immunizations. In the 1980s, the Universal Childhood Immunization (UCI) resulted in the establishment of national systems of immunization and rapidly rising immunization coverage. Thanks to the establishment of strong immunization services over two-thirds of the world's targeted population is now reached with immunizations. As a result, more than two million deaths from vaccine preventable diseases (VPD) were prevented in 2002, and 600 000 liver cirrhosis and hepatoma deaths from hepatitis B will be prevented in the future due to vaccination efforts in that year.

Immunization against infectious diseases is one of the key inventions of the last century and biggest successes of modern medicine. Perhaps no other human endeavour has had as dramatic, deep and positive legacy as immunization. Of global deaths among children, less than five years of age, a significant proportion dies of vaccine preventable diseases. These include 770,000 deaths due to measles and 200,000 deaths due to neonatal tetanus. Many of these children are already otherwise compromised by malnutrition or other infectious diseases. In a country like India, by vaccinating 1000 infants we can prevent about 30 deaths from measles and 10 deaths from whooping cough. Vaccinating 1000 women with tetanus toxoid (TT) prevents five deaths from neonatal tetanus. Immunization is one of the most cost-effective public health interventions available. Yet, a large proportion of vulnerable infants and children in India are not receiving this simple intervention. Across India in 2001-02, only 63.6 per cent of children 12-23 months had received all six of their primary vaccines, with a wide variation among states. States with poorer immunization rates generally have higher child mortality rates. A successful immunization programme is an indication of a strong and functioning public health system.

The material and human progress so many societies have made

rests heavily on public health improvements of which immunization is a linchpin. Yet it does not receive the attention and acclaim it deserves even in the developing world. Since 1970, global coverage has soared from less than 10 per cent to almost 75 per cent in 2003 and saving 2.5 million children every year—a towering achievement by any means.

Issues and Challenges for the Millennium Development Goals (MDGs)[3]

Achieving high immunization coverage and sustaining it is one of the main challenges for the MDG when coverage data indicates that performance is slipping back. The frontline strategy should be to reach the unreached and accelerate disease control efforts—polio eradication, NNT elimination and measles control.

Vaccines have changed the future course of history and human development and they continue to do so. Relatively recent vaccines and vaccine delivery technologies hold enormous promise but the unacceptable reality is that many in the developing countries will continue to be excluded from their benefits. A vaccine now offers protection against hepatitis B (causing liver cancer later in life). Then there is Hib vaccine (Haemophilus influenzae type B causing bacterial pneumonia and meningitis) which has been introduced in 24 developing countries. At least 400,000 children die every year from the infections of Hib causes. Pneumococcal vaccine was licensed last year for use in USA. More than half of the pneumonia deaths are attributable to this infection. Yellow fever vaccine, though available for the past 65 years, is not reachable for many who need it routinely. Rotavirus vaccine can prevent one quarter of the 1.8 million children deaths every year. Vaccines are also being developed for dysentery and E.coli infections each of which kill upwards of five lakh children every year. Malaria and HIV/AIDs vaccine are under research and could be available in the next five to ten years. Other vaccines being tested are for diseases such as schistosomiasis and dengue, which infect millions of children and adults, every year. Implementation of these new vaccines will be a major issue.

Preventing disease through immunization benefits all people, resulting in positive health, economic and social yield at global, national and community levels. Immunization is a cost-effective and life-saving intervention, preventing needless diseases, disabilities and deaths. In the current context of globalization, acting together against childhood communicable diseases that are preventable by vaccines and preparing for the possible emergence of diseases with pandemic potential will contribute significantly to the enhancement of global health and security.

Immunization and other linked interventions as described in this document will provide an important contribution to achieving the Millennium Development Goals (MDGs) either directly by contributing to the reduction of childhood deaths or indirectly in reducing the incidence of other infectious diseases, and, ultimately, by improving the health of the population and thus contributing to poverty reduction.

Immunization in India

Vaccination was practised in India since the early 1900s, especially against small-pox, in the late 1940's. In 1962, BCG inoculation was included in the National Tuberculosis Control Programme. A formal programme under the name of Expanded Programme of Immunization (EPI) was launched in 1978. This gained momentum in 1985 under UIP. The main objectives of this programme were universal immunization, reduction in mortality and morbidity due to VPDs, achievement of self-sufficiency in vaccine production, establishment of a cold chain system and introduction of a district level monitoring system. UIP was merged in child survival and safe motherhood programme (CSSM) in 1992-93. Since 1997 immunization activities are an important component of the national RCH programme. A National Technical Advisory Group on Immunization (NTAGI) was set up in 2003 and a Mid-term Strategic Plan (MTSP) developed in 2004. From April 2005 immunization is an important component of Reproductive and Child Health Programme (RCH II) under the National Rural Health Mission (NRHM).

In the last 15-20 years, several feats have been achieved globally and in India. NNT has been eliminated from 111 countries while 160 countries are polio-free. In India, 20 districts are polio-endemic and one-third of the districts endemic for NNT. Globally, mortality and morbidity caused by measles declined by 86 per cent and 74 per cent respectively. In India, measles morbidity reduced by 82 per cent and mortality by 70 per cent. The experience with polio, while filling us with satisfaction, must also drive us to consolidate our accomplishments by turning the power of immunization on diseases that are still killing millions of children and impairing the abilities of countless others. Just as a new generation of vaccines capable of saving million more children's lives each year is about to come in the market, maybe, at a greater cost—the momentum to sustain immunization is faltering.

Immunization Coverage

The percentage of children receiving the final dose of DPT3 reveals how well countries or states are providing immunization coverage for their children. The world average for DPT3 in 1999 was 77 per cent. In India the reported coverage of DPT3 has been between 89 and 95 per cent since 1990. The nation's reported coverage for each antigen since 1990 has increased, with the exceptions of 1992 and 2001. BCG coverage rates have been over 100 per cent for the last three years (perhaps due to an under-estimation of the denominator). The reported national BCG—measles dropout rate is 10 per cent in 2002.

The evaluated coverage was declining from 77 per cent in 1996-97 to 47 per cent in 1999-00. However, in 2000-01, coverage increased to 63.6 per cent (CES-01-02, UNICEF). Interstate variation is significant (Figure 1).

Variations between districts: In 1998-99 GOI started organizing Rapid Household Surveys (RHS) of basic indicators. So far two rounds have been completed. Figure 3 shows the evaluated district-wise RCH fully immunized coverage surveys comparing 1998-99 and 2002-03. This not only emphasizes the low coverage rates in districts within the northern States, but also helps identify areas of poorer performance lying within states with higher average coverage rates.

Of the 260, 176 (72 per cent) districts surveyed showed a decrease in full immunization rates over five years: average decrease 15.4 per cent (range 0.1 - 64.2 per cent)

66 (27 per cent) districts showed an increase in full immunization rates over five years; average increase 9.4 per cent (varied 0.1 - 41.1 per cent). Two districts showed no change in full immunization rates.

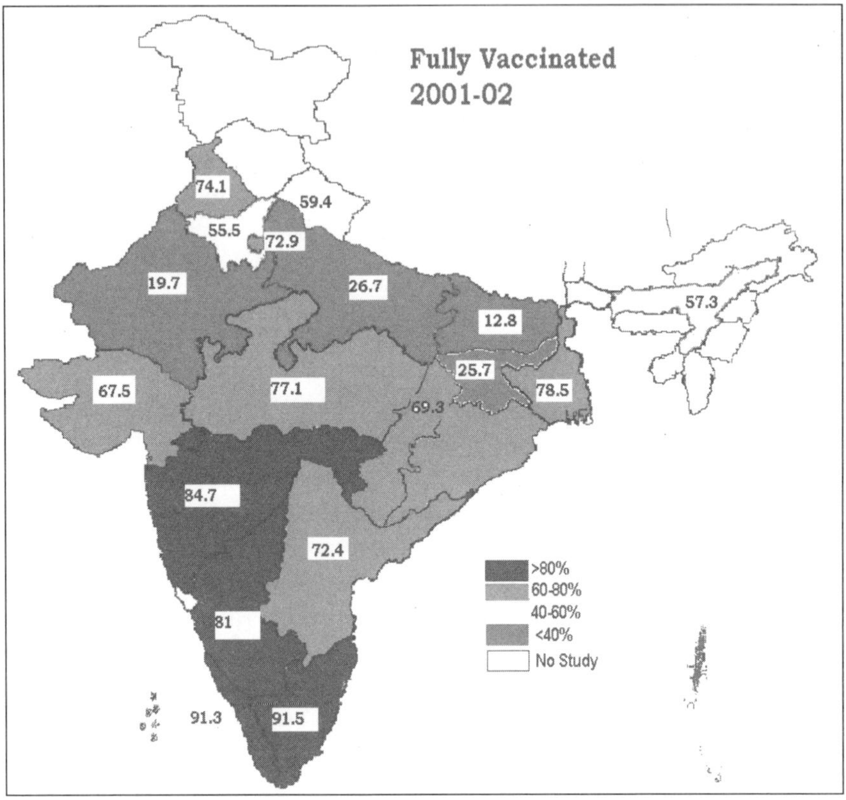

Figure 1

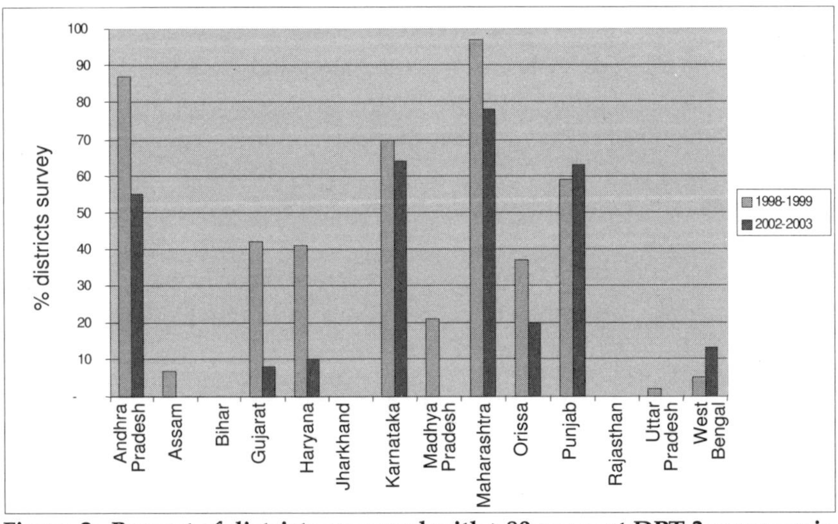

Figure 2: Percent of districts surveyed with >80 per cent DPT 3 coverage in key States in 1998-99 and 2002-03[4] Source: Rapid Household Survey RCH project; International Institute for Population Sciences

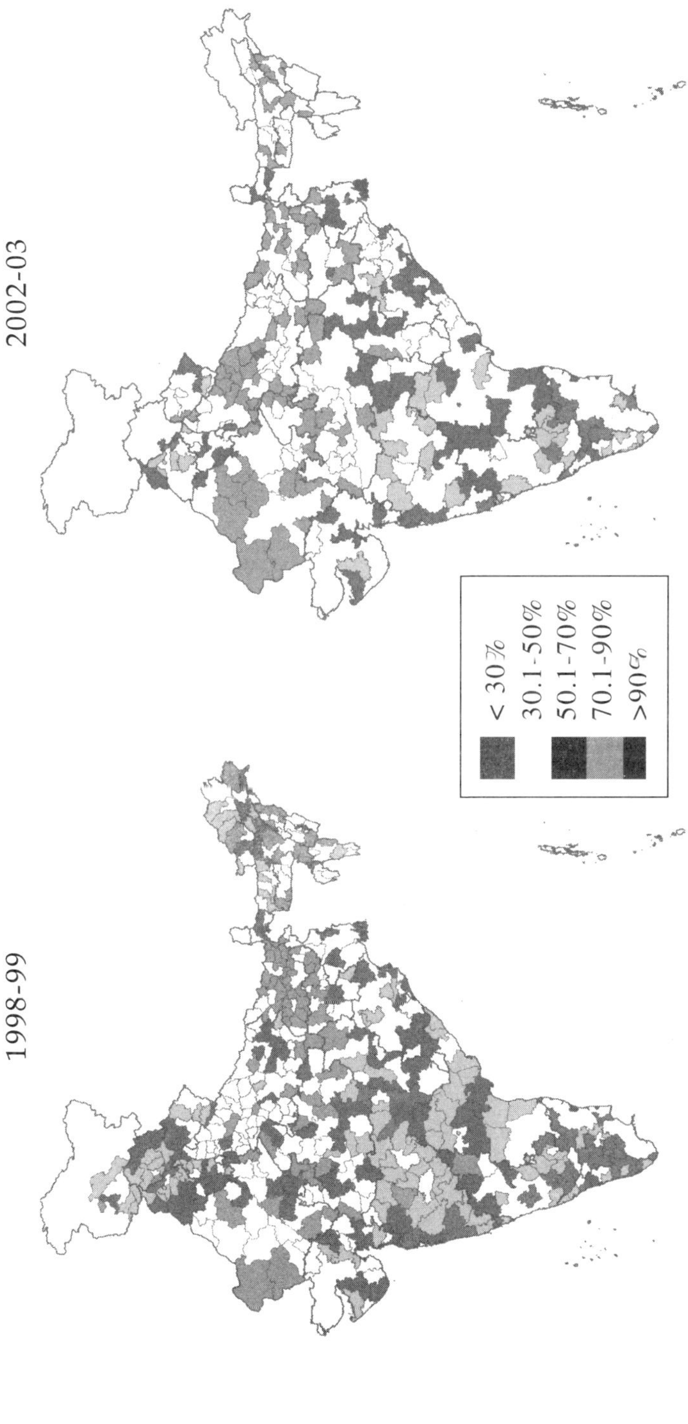

Figure 3: Evaluated fully immunized coverage rate, by district, comparing 1998-99 survey with 2002-03 (260 districts). Source: Rapid Household Survey RCH project; International Institute for Population Sciences.

Dropout Rate

In India we looked at the dropout rates between highest covered antigen (BCG generally) and measles. Statewise the BCG-DPT3 dropout rates varied between 10-40 per cent in 2001, and overall 14.4 per cent. The dropout rate is an indicator of acceptability or demand for immunization services. **Almost 6.3 million children who came into contact with immunization services (receiving BCG) in 2001 did not receive their measles vaccine.** Ninety-three per cent of these infants live in 15 states and over half live in Andhra Pradesh, Uttar Pradesh, West Bengal and Bihar. These spell bad news for the health of young children and present a challenge for local health delivery systems. The figures show that caregivers had been in contact with service providers because they had received the BCG shot. They did not, however, return with their children to receive three doses of DPT. They were either dissatisfied with the services or were not even made aware that a complete course was needed. Data indicates that overall 72.8 per cent of the children are reached and dropout is around 14.4 per cent.

Situational Analysis[5]

As mentioned above, research findings for the period 1996-97 to March-May 2001 indicate that immunization coverage levels have declined over the past 5-6 years (Figure 4).

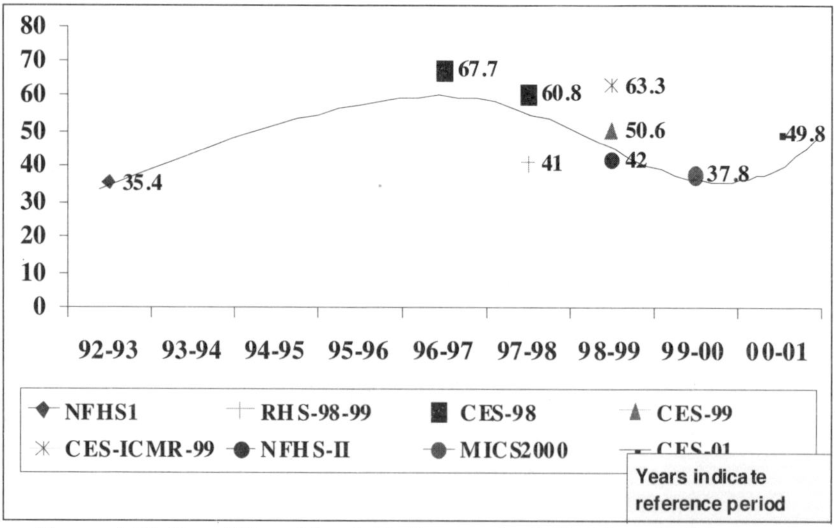

Figure 4: National Trend for Fully Immunized Children (All Surveys)

Evidence also indicates that coverage levels are significantly higher in those areas with regular access to the services (63 per cent) as compared to those communities where sessions are less frequent or irregular (33 per cent).

Routine reporting is currently complemented by periodical coverage evaluation surveys that offer updated information. The data indicates that DPT3 reported coverage was 89 per cent in 2000 (MoHFW, GOI) while it was only 63.6 per cent as per the CES-2001 results. Contrary to routine reporting, the 2000-01 DPT3 gap refers to 7 million fewer children under one year of age that have missed DPT3. The discrepancy in the number estimated is more evident in Uttar Pradesh, Bihar, Madhya Pradesh, Orissa and Rajasthan.

The following graph depicts the evaluated coverage of routine immunization in the northern states between 1998-2002. An analysis of the trends demonstrates that West Bengal, Madhya Pradesh and Uttaranchal experienced a rise in coverage, while Bihar stagnated at a low of 12 per cent. Delhi underwent a rise to 70 per cent in 2000-2001 that was not sustained in 2002 as coverage dropped to approximately 65 per cent.

In general, as recently outlined by the Department of Family Welfare (DFW) in its call to accelerate routine immunization in the northern states, reported coverage rates are typically higher—sometimes double those estimated by the surveys. Four of the 10 states have state-wide coverage greater than 50 per cent (Gujarat, Chhattisgarh, Orissa and West Bengal), but none of the ten states

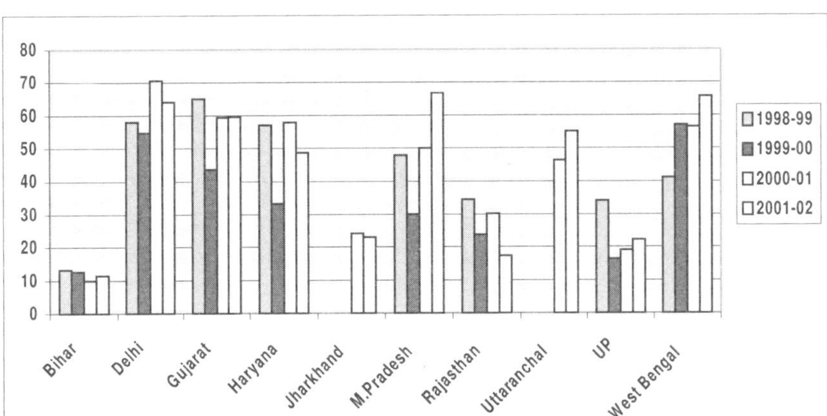

Figure 5: Evaluated Coverage of RI in the Northern States between 1998-2002

has achieved coverage higher than 29 per cent in their lowest coverage district. Cold chain equipment has been imported but technical assistance is lacking. The reliability and continuity of power supply are also identified as a major system problems for adequate vaccine management and cash to comply with fuel for generators sets represents a major state drawback in Uttar Pradesh, Bihar, Jharkhand and West Bengal.

It has become apparent that unless routine immunization services are strengthened or accelerated in all these states as a matter of urgency, there will be a generalized re-occurrence of diphtheria and pertussis, as well as measles foci. Furthermore, Hepatitis B vaccine will be available to no more than 5 per cent to 30 per cent of the children in the lowest coverage areas. Hence the opportunity to widely introduce the GAVI-funded Hepatitis B vaccine will be missed

Reported coverage has remained high since 1990. But, national coverage reports of over 100 per cent show that there are problems with the accuracy of reported coverage. Therefore, coverage surveys are routinely used to evaluate coverage of the vaccines.

Despite only fully protecting about half of all infants, infant mortality rate (IMR) declined during the phasing in of the UIP, especially in 1990 when national coverage was achieved (Figure 6). IMR continued to decline after 1990. The Child Survival Safe Motherhood (CSSM) and Reproductive Child Health (RCH) programmes started in 1992 and 1997, respectively, included the UIP as a key component, and built upon the infrastructure developed for the UIP. The IMR in India remains high. It is likely that strengthening routine immunization would reduce the IMR, and thus have a large impact on the global total of childhood deaths.

The UIP protects infants against six vaccine preventable diseases. (Hepatitis B vaccine is being progressively added to the UIP with national coverage planned by 2009). Every year, the UIP protects more infants against these diseases than any other in the world, with the possible exception of China. The resultant decline in the diseases is shown in Figure 7.

India also has the largest number of infants who reach their first birthday not fully immunized. (Estimated at nearly 18 million for the 2001 birth cohort). Surveillance quality tends to be worst in areas with lowest coverage. So, reported diseases represent only a small fraction of actual disease incidence—except for polio that is nearly

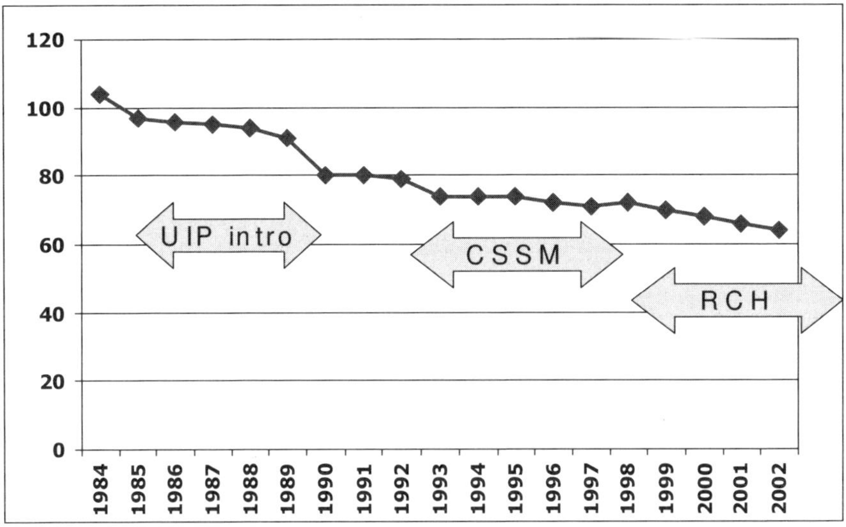

Figure 6: National Infant Mortality Rate per 1000 Live Births, 1984 to 2002

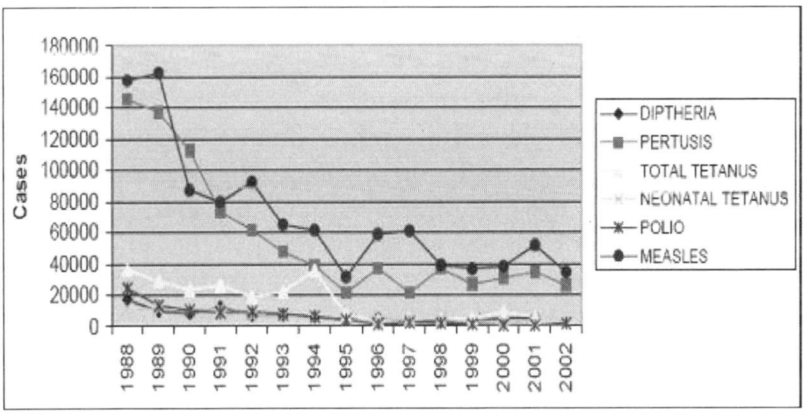

Figure 7: Reported Cases of UIP diseases[6]

eliminated from the National Polio Surveillance Programme (NPSP) and Pulse Polio Immunization (PPI).

Despite these problems, incidence of UIP diseases has substantially decreased since 1985. But, much work remains to protect all of India's children from these preventable diseases. The size and diversity of India make this especially challenging, as do resource constraints and competing priorities. The UIP has developed a multi-year plan (MYP) for 2004 to 2009 that aims to address these challenges.

Why Are We Not Achieving Higher Immunization Coverage Rates?

There are several reasons that have been put forward for poor immunization rates, both globally and in the Indian context. The main reasons for the low immunization rates and poor vaccine effectiveness as identified by the National Family Health Survey 1998-99 (NFHS-II) and the qualitative surveys are the following:

- Inadequate delivery of health services (supply shortages, vacant staff positions, lack of training).
- Poor maintenance of the cold chain.
- Inadequate supervision and monitoring of the programme.
- Weak surveillance for all vaccine preventable diseases except polio.
- Injection safety not assured.
- No provision made for medical waste disposal.
- General lack of inter-sectoral coordination, resulting in missing opportunities to improve immunization coverage and quality.
- Date, place, and time of immunization sessions varied, making it difficult for parents to access services.
- Inadequate technical capacities among service providers, such as a lack of clarity on proper methods of reconstitution of vaccines, and the administration of intradermal injections.
- Complacency, for several reasons such as the belief that since some disease are not common they are not important, or a mistaken belief that measles is common and therefore not a dangerous disease.
- Lack of support for ANMs from other staff at the health centres.
- Lack of updated information, education and communication (IEC) materials.
- Parental non-acceptance of immunization due to various reasons (Fig. 8).
- Lack of information/awareness of day/time/place of immunization sessions.
- Lack of awareness of the importance of/need for immunization.
- No one available to take a child to the sessions.
- Lack of faith in immunization.

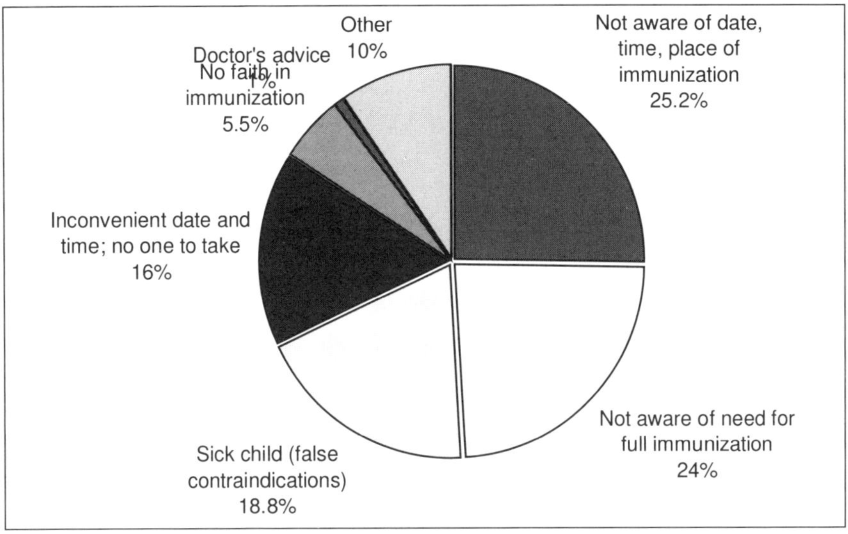

Figure 8: Reasons for Low Coverage

It is clear from the above list that the problem lies at various levels in the system, including planning, training, implementation and monitoring of the programme. Some of these relate to inadequate resources; some to inadequate use of available resources; either due to poor knowledge and training or due to inadequate management systems. This section will attempt to fill the information gaps and to provide rational basis for strengthening the operational aspects of the programme.

Where are the un-immunized? 17.9 million infants were not fully immunized in India in 2001-2, which represents about a third of the global total. Ninety-five per cent of these unimmunized infants live in 15 States; 40 per cent live in Uttar Pradesh and Bihar.

Injection Safety and Unsafe Waste Disposal

A recent INCLEN study demonstrated that 73.9 per cent of injections given in the immunization programme were deemed to be unsafe (of this 27.1percent due to questionable sterility, 15.2 per cent reuse and 65.5 per cent due to wrong habit). WHO estimates that in the South East Asia Region unsafe injections contribute to 31 per cent of new cases of HIV, 59 per cent of Hepatitis B and 92 per cent of Hepatitis C. In India out of 25 million infants born every year, over 1 million run the lifetime risk of developing chronic hepatitis B virus infection. This worrying trend is highlighted in the plan and the GoI is committed to address the issue. The most important development of 2004 in this regard was the announcement on the floor of the Parliament the introduction of auto-disable syringes countrywide from April 2005.

Vaccine Production

In 20 years, India has developed its capacity to manufacture all vaccines except OPV. However, quality including General Manufacturing Practices (GMP) needs to be monitored continuously as is being done for polio vaccine. OPV potency testing is done before releasing. In 1999-2000, vaccine vial monitors were introduced on polio vaccine vials to monitor the quality of vaccine in field. No such monitor is available for other vaccines as yet.

The Immunological Basis of Immunization

Immunization is based on the principle that if the body is exposed in a controlled manner to infective agents, it develops the capacity to fight infections in future. This ability is the immunity status of the body against specific infection, and functions on the inherent ability of the body to recognize, fight and memorise its actions against an infective agent.

How does a Vaccine Protect an Individual Child?

A vaccine contains an antigen, such as bacteria or virus or part of the organism that is capable of provoking an immune response in the body. Upon administering the vaccine, there is an immune response in the body similar to that of the original microbe. The vaccine, however, does not cause the disease, and the immune response to the antigen protects the body from any invasion by such a microbe in the future.

Multi-Year Plan for UIP, 2004-09[7]

The context for the MYP includes immunization specific goals of the National Population Policy 2000, in the National Socio-Demographic Goals for 2010:

- Reduce infant mortality rate to below 30 per 1000 live births.
- Achieve universal immunization of children against all vaccine preventable diseases.

UIP Mission Statement

To provide high quality immunization services to all communities in order to prevent mortality, morbidity and disability from diseases that are preventable through the optimum use of vaccines that are currently available and vaccines that become available from time to time.

The four essential elements for achieving the desired child protection goals would be:

1. **Facilitating development of new and improved vaccines.** This involves: (i) developing consensus on priority new vaccines and the improvement of existing ones; (ii) acquiring epidemiological and economic data on infectious diseases to guide decision-making; (iii) Promoting research and development efforts on new vaccines, those using combination methodologies, and/or vaccines based on new technologies; (iv) developing oral and other mucosally-delivered vaccines which are easy to administer and provide better protection than injectable ones against pathogens entering the body via mucosal surfaces; and (v) promotion of more thermostable vaccines which are free from adverse reactions and harmonize vaccine delivery schedules.

2. **Promoting the wide availability of quality vaccines.** This involves encouraging governments to establish National Control Authorities (NCA), enhancing local efforts to improve vaccine quality, ensuring availability of reference materials to assure quality, and fostering communication among NCAs, regulatory bodies and other organizations interested in vaccine quality. It also involves encouraging governments towards self-sufficiency, adequate financing of immunization programmes, creating and expanding demand for vaccines, and planning to provide vaccines supply in emergencies.

3. **Promoting the introduction and use of needed vaccines.** This includes the promotion, selection and introduction of priority new vaccines in national immunization programmes and promoting safety of injection practices. It encompasses encouraging the collection of reliable information on which to base estimates of the burden and costs of infectious diseases of local relevance for national decision-making. It also calls for support to social and behavioural research designed to foster a better understanding of factors leading

to increased societal acceptance and use of vaccines. It might also mean promoting access of the under-reached/unreached groups of populations to national delivery systems and vaccines, encouraging innovative approaches to improving distribution and delivery of vaccines, and fostering methods to encourage community participation and gender equality.

4. Fostering a culture of prevention through advocacy for vaccines: This involves increasing awareness of the demand for vaccines, disease elimination/eradication through vaccination and disease surveillance and mobilizing the resources needed.

UIP Guiding Principles to Achieve its Mission

(a) **Maximal reach**: to overcome barriers at all levels, to sustain demand and ensure all pregnant mothers and children are immunized as per the national schedule

(b) **Equity**: aiming to reduce disparities in services by addressing the needs of the under served

(c) **Quality and safety**: the immunization programme will follow recommended practices in vaccine procurement, storage, distribution and service delivery

(d) **Sustainability**: ensuring sufficient financial and human resources for long-term needs for immunization services, through investments by GoI and key partners

(e) **Management excellence**: The UIP, in collaboration with key partner agencies and professional organizations, will optimize the use of resources following result-based principles and evidence-based practices.

The medium term plan envisions six goals, each with its own set of objectives, strategies to reach those objectives and indicators to measure progress:

GOAL 1 - Districts provide efficient and safe immunization services to all infants and pregnant women

GOAL 2 - Contribute to global polio eradication, measles mortality reduction and NNT elimination

GOAL 3 - Have sufficient and sustainable funding and established adequate, accountable and efficient fund flows

GOAL 4 - There is sustained demand and reduced social barriers to access immunization services

GOAL 5 - Accelerated introduction of licensed new and underutilized vaccines against diseases with significant mortality and morbidity in India

GOAL 6 - To monitor and use accurate, complete and timely data on vaccine preventable diseases, AEFIs and antigen coverage and dropout rates by district

Immunization and other linked interventions as described in this document will provide an important contribution to achieving the Millennium Development Goals (MDGs) either directly by contributing to the reduction of childhood deaths or indirectly in reducing the incidence of other infectious diseases, and ultimately, by improving the health of the population and thus contributing to poverty reduction. Specific goals that may benefit from widespread immunization include:

- Reduce child mortality by two-thirds between 1990 and 2015 (Goal 4) with the indicator of the proportion of one-year-old children immunized against measles;
- Improve maternal health by reducing by three quarters the maternal mortality ratio (Goal 5), and
- Combat HIV/AIDS, malaria and other diseases (Goal 6) by halting and beginning to reverse the incidence of malaria and other major diseases.

The Global Alliance for Vaccines and Immunizations (GAVI) has set milestones for selective immunization goals.[8] These include:

- By 2010, 90 per cent coverage for all children in all countries and 80 per cent coverage in all districts;
- By 2007, hepatitis B vaccines introduced in all countries with adequate delivery systems; and
- By 2005, Hib vaccine introduced into 50 per cent of the poorest countries with the highest disease burden.

Vision

We strive for a world in 2015 where:

- Immunization is highly valued
- Every child, adolescent and adult will have equal access to immunization as provided for in the national schedule
- More people are protected against more diseases

Guiding Principles

The following guiding principles have inspired the formulation of the GIVS:

Equity and gender equality: All people—independent of their socio-cultural, economic, gender and geographic specificities—should have equal access to the needed vaccines and interventions.

Ownership, partnership and responsibility: Joined by international solidarity, governments and their partners pursue common agreed goals and engage in coordinated activities determined by national plans.

Accountability: Stakeholders and actors in immunization are publicly accountable for their policies and actions.

Quality products and services: All products made available meet internationally recognized standards of quality and services are delivered according to best practices.

Strong district-based immunization systems: The focus of interventions and their monitoring at district level ensure local commitment and ownership and the appropriate adaptation of the programme to local needs and circumstances.

Sustainability through technical and financial capacity building: National governments and partners should collectively strive for financial and technical self-reliance and incremental infrastructure building on an ongoing basis.

Policies and strategies based on evidence and best practices: Operational research, data from monitoring and evaluation systems, disease burden and impact assessments, economic analysis, lessons from other countries in similar circumstances and experiences inform the choice of strategies and practices.

Immunization has saved the lives of millions of children in the three decades since the launch of the Expanded Programme on Immunization (EPI) in 1974. Yet over 27 million children below the age of one and 40 million pregnant women worldwide are still overlooked by routine immunization services. As a result, vaccine-preventable diseases are estimated to cause more than two million deaths every year. It is expected that improvements and cost reductions in the current vaccines will make them available in the near future to all children who need them. The effectiveness of immunization is thoroughly proven. Unlike most other health and development interventions, immunization does not simply raise the chances that children will resist a disease: it virtually guarantees they will. Each year since 1990, routine immunization with vaccine against diphtheria, pertussis and tetanus has reached more than 70 per cent of all children, an extraordinary accomplishment considering that more than 130 million children are born each year and need to be immunized. Combined with accelerated disease control programmes, routine services have contributed significantly to child survival, averting more than two million deaths a year and preventing countless episodes of illness and disability.

Disease surveillance, injection safety which includes safe injection practice, reduction in injection overuse, availability of adequate and quality injection equipment and safe management of sharps and plastics and quality of vaccine needs to be addressed before expecting quality improvement in routine immunization.

REFERENCES

1. Immunization and Vaccine Preventable Diseases, Care.
2. Coverage Evaluation Survey 2001-02, Government of India.
3. Millennium Development Goals, www.who.int.
4. Rapid Household Survey, International Institute of Population Sciences, Mumbai, India.
5. Immunization Plus, A Framework for Action 2003-2007, UNICEF, India, May 2003.
6. Reported cases of VPDs, Central Bureau of Health Intelligence, Government of India.
7. Multi Year Plan of Government of India.
8. Global Immunization Vision and Strategies (GIVS), A Strategic Framework for 2006-15.

3

Vaccination Programmes: Limitations as a Universal Solution

Dr. Rajib Dasgupta

Introduction

Infectious diseases are occupying centrestage with SARS, Japanese Encephalitis (JE) and Avian Influenza dominating the public discourse. Wherever possible, vaccines are being chosen as the preferred option. Following the Japanese encephalitis epidemic in Uttar Pradesh, efforts are on to initiate JE vaccination programme under the Universal Immunisation Programme (UIP) in a campaign mode with intense social mobilisation. An effective AIDS vaccine is a social hope and a technological aspiration. A trial is being conducted by a partnership between the Government of India—through the Indian Council of Medical Research (ICMR) and the National AIDS Control Organization (NACO)—and the not-for-profit International AIDS Vaccine Initiative (IAVI). Current campaigns have hailed immunisation as the 'one' or 'universal' solution for a range of infectious diseases. This is being advocated under the banner of the National Rural Health Mission (NRHM) and international agencies like UNICEF have intensified their commitment. While vaccines are an oft prescribed public health solution to several infectious diseases, they are not without problems. The paper examines key issues of largescale vaccination through the two most recent and popular programmes—Hepatitis B and Oral Polio Vaccines.

This paper is a systematic review of the considerable volume of work that exists in the context of the two recent high-profile vaccination programmes—Hepatitis B and the Global Polio Eradication Initiative (GPEI) popularly referred to as the Pulse Polio campaign. This paper initially starts with a short review of McKeown's thesis analysing the role of specific medical measures including vaccination in control of communicable diseases. This debate has recently been reopened. In the context of Hepatitis B and Polio, the review has attempted to triangulate three elements—the epidemiology of the disease, the epidemiologic rationale of the programmes and the political and economic forces that have shaped these programmes.

I. McKeown's Argument

How far have vaccines been responsible for the decline of infectious diseases in the developed nations? McKeown and Record (1992) analysed mortality data for nineteenth century England and Wales in order to explore the trends in demographic changes. They demonstrated that two-thirds of the reduction in mortality during the first half of the century could be explained by decline in deaths from infectious diseases. They attributed the decline of infections to one or more of the three groups of factors:

- medical measures of preventing and treating disease in the individual.
- a spontaneous decline in mortality.
- a heterogeneous group of factors referred to collectively as improvements in the environment.

There is little doubt that till 1935, there were no specific medical measures or technology available to account for the spectacular decline. Microbes for most infectious diseases were not identified till the last quarter of the nineteenth century. Medical measures were thus considered to contribute very little to the decline of mortality till the 1930s. They further argued that though a spontaneous change in the relation between the infective agent and the human host accounted for deaths from diseases like scarlet fever, it was unlikely to have affected decline in mortality from major causes such as tuberculosis or cholera.

The most significant contribution was made by two kinds of improvement in the environment—a rising standard of living, particularly, improved diet, and, hygienic changes introduced by the sanitary reformers. There was a large reduction of mortality from TB when the standard of living and diet improved at a time when neither any medical measure was available nor any reduction in the virulence of the bacillus was demonstrated. Current opinions state that McKeown over-estimated the mortality gains from reduction from TB. Intestinal infections declined when public health legislation led to significant improvements in water supplies and sewage disposal. The arguments about better food availability and nutrition have been criticised on grounds of lack of evidence and McKeown himself had acknowledged the weakness of that argument. However, the basic argument about medical interventions and declines in infectious diseases essentially remains valid (Grundy, 2005).

II. The Case of the Hepatitis B Vaccine

The Union Ministry of Health and Family Welfare announced inclusion of the Hepatitis B vaccine in the Universal Immunisation Programme on September 5, 2005. The Union Health Minister was quoted as saying, "Hepatitis B has reached alarming levels and is increasing every year. That's why we have decided to bring this vaccine under our National Immunisation Programme. The vaccine will now be administered in combination with DPTs to all children in their 4th, 6th and 12th week from 2006. We have been carrying out clinical trials of this combination across 15 cities and 32 districts and it has proved highly effective. The problem has become bigger even than AIDS' (*Times of India*, 2005). In the same report, Health Ministry officials were quoted as saying that the country has the world's second largest pool of carriers of the lethal disease—43 million—out of whom 10 per cent were highly infectious.

The 'clinical trials' referred to above was actually a pilot project that was launched in 2002 by the then Prime Minister with the long-term plan to expand it to the entire country during the Tenth Plan (*The Hindu*, 2002). The World Health Organisation (WHO, 1995) prescribed the universal immunisation strategy; this evolved from the earlier positions of selective immunisation to high-risk groups and then universal immunisation for countries with high endemicity. Despite the WHO's position, several European countries, including the United Kingdom, did not implement the strategy citing low endemicity (in their populations) and high cost of the vaccine

(Damme, 1996 and CLDF, 2005). In the Indian context, suitable strategies for the public health management of this problem are being intensely debated (Dasgupta, 2005, Aggarwal, 2004 and Sahni et al, 2004).

Hepatitis B is transmitted through diverse routes—sexual, needles, transplacental and blood and blood products. The clinicians have been arguing for decades that HB is a problem of far greater importance than HIV/AIDS, and rightly so. Despite a range of pressing public health problems crying for attention, it is interesting that HIV/AIDS has become a gold-standard for epidemiological ranking of diseases—not because the disease is highly prevalent but because the political backing and funds that it attracts. Despite close similarity in transmission with HIV/AIDS the 'high-risk' approach was initially adopted for Hepatitis B with regard to vaccines but not so for 'lifestyles'. There were no major systemic approaches to correct ills in the healthcare delivery system. While social sciences research in HIV/AIDS led to the adoption of a range of interventions the availability of the Hepatitis B vaccine led to the invocation of the germ theory paradigm. Statements like 'eradication of HBV worldwide is a distinct possibility' just because, 'fortunately, there are very effective vaccines against the virus, which are about 95 per cent effective' published in as leading a journal as *Lancet* show complete lack of understanding of epidemiological complexities—both of disease transmission and health services (Lai, 2003).

Claims about numbers are largely based on hospital centred studies that use HBsAg sero-prevalence as an indicator; point prevalence studies cannot be extrapolated as indicative of the total load in the community. HBsAg and HBeAg rates vary widely in different states and regions of the country. Community-based studies suggest that while jaundice is associated with about one per cent of all causes of deaths, symptoms suggestive of chronic liver disease including cirrhosis are reported to be responsible for only about 0.76 per cent of total deaths. The epidemiological logic for immunisation against Hepatitis B is that if the infection is acquired in infancy or childhood there is a higher probability of chronic liver disease later in adult life that in turn could lead to hepatocellular carcinoma, cirrhosis, liver failure and death. Mohandas (2000) argued on the basis of data available through cancer registries and migrant studies that hepatocellular carcinoma (accounting for only 1.6 per cent of all cancer deaths) certainly was not prevalent in India to the extent of many South-East Asian countries. Phadke (2000) estimated that the HBsAg carrier rate in India was about 1.42 per cent of the general population and the carrier pool about 12.75 million (considerably lower than the official estimate of 43 million computed on the basis of 4.2 per cent average prevalence across the country). The HBeAg pool was computed to be only 3.26 million implying that only 3.1 per cent of chronic hepatitis B carriers would die of liver diseases in contrast to the oft-quoted figure of 25 per cent. By these estimates, less than 0.1 per cent of new-borns would die of the sequelae of Hepatitis B infection in their lifetime compared to the average infant mortality of seven per cent.

What are the implications for the inclusion of this vaccine in the UIP? Universal infant immunisation leads to rapid reduction of the transmission from mother to child, or from child to child within the first year wherever prevalence of HBsAg is greater than eight per cent. Tamil Nadu, Andhra Pradesh, Madhya Pradesh and Uttar Pradesh have a prevalence of >4 per cent zone. For populations with intermediate endemicity (HBsAg prevalence 2–4 per cent) and low endemicity (HBsAg prevalence <2 per cent) substantial disease burden has been attributed to chronic infections acquired by older children, adolescents and adults; catch-up strategies have been advised for cohorts such as adolescents and persons with risk factors for acquiring hepatitis B viral infection, in addition to routine infant vaccination (http://www.who.int/vaccines, 2004 and http://www.who.int/emc, 2004). Karnataka, Maharashtra, Delhi, Haryana, Himachal Pradesh and West Bengal have reported prevalence rate of 2-4 per cent and the other states lower (Mohandas, 2000). A universal immunisation strategy across the country without catch-up strategies (since most of our states have intermediate or low endemicity) is clearly not going to make an impact despite huge commitment of resources.

Currently suggested vaccination schedules include three options with two of them including a dose at birth; in populations where a lower proportion of chronic infections are acquired perinatally, priority should be accorded to achieve high DPT3 and HB3 vaccine coverage among infants. In order to reduce transmission from mother to baby, the first dose needs to be administered as soon as possible after birth and certainly within 24 hours (http://www.who.int/

vaccines, 2004 and http://www.who.int/emc, 2004). The Indian programme has recently included a zero-day dose, that is, administering the vaccine within the first 24 hours of birth. But, as has been argued later, the reach of the zero-day vaccine will be limited. It is synchronised with three doses of DPT vaccine based on the argument that in low HBeAg prevalence situations the vaccine is as effective if delivered with the DPT vaccine. HBeAg rates in pregnant women in India have wide variations across states/regions (reported range 7.8 to 47.8 per cent, mean 24.01percent) and there is no justification in assuming that HBeAg positivity among Indian mothers is 'low'. Chronicity of the infection, which is the driving force for universal immunisation, is age-related; children aged less than a year have 90 per cent risk of chronicity; the risk reduces to about 30 per cent for children aged one to five years and about two per cent for adults (Hyams, 1995).

Dasgupta and Priya (2002) estimated the efficiency of the vaccine delivery on the basis of available data from the National Family Health Survey (NFHS). The potential for delivery of a zero-day dose based on institutional and assisted deliveries was estimated to range from 20 per cent to 45 per cent for major Indian states; going by the actual delivery of the zero-day dose of the high-profile polio vaccine, the figure was about 13 per cent (range 2 to 11 per cent), except Kerala and Tamil Nadu for both these variables. If it is delivered with the DPT, the coverage of the crucial third dose was estimated nationally to be about 55 per cent. What is of concern is the decline of DPT3 coverage in crucial states like Bihar, Madhya Pradesh, Rajasthan and Uttar Pradesh between the two rounds of the NFHS. In the past few years there is increasing recognition and concern that routine immunisation coverage has declined owing to over-emphasis on the polio eradication programme (Planning Commission, Tenth Plan, undated). The number of paediatric doses of Hepatitis B vaccines required annually to fully cover the estimated infant population for 2002-06 was estimated to be 62.6-79.5 million doses, assuming zero wastage. While production capacities are adequate for DPT and OPV, Hepatitis B vaccine will need to be imported.

This has significant implications for the cost and sustainability of the programme. In the context of the Hepatitis B vaccine, Madhavi (2003) has analysed in detail the market forces, the nature of negotiations between the state and the private players and the role being played by the Global Alliance for Vaccines and Immunisation (GAVI) in great detail. It is also understood that India will be implementing the programme initially through large loans and will have to find resources internally in due course. A recent instance of misuse of state powers to promote the vaccine was a directive in January 2004 from the then Minister of State, Human Resources Development, himself an onco-surgeon, that teachers, students and staff of all University Grants Commission institutions and colleges should be immunised with the Hepatitis B vaccine; however, this was not implemented (Dasgupta, 2005).

Recent WHO directives of using the Auto Disabled (AD) syringes for immunisation and the Government of India's implementation plans will push up the cost of this component by about three times. The norms of proper disposal of such huge quantities of plastic demand a level of rigour that would be hard to attain in the peripheral institutions. All current EPI vaccines require 11.0 cm^3 of storage space per dose. Inclusion of monovalent HB vaccine would require augmentation of storage (cold chain) capacity by about 25 per cent, on a nation-wide scale. The October 2004 document of the Government of India on Infection Management and Environment Plan (IMEP) for the Reproductive and Child Health Programme, Phase II (GoI, 2004) stated that AD syringes will be introduced in a phased manner in RCH-II. Two hundred and eighty million of AD syringes will be used per annum, implying that almost 2150 tonnes of plastics, 613 tonnes of needles and 20 tonnes of glass waste need to be disposed per annum.

The relative high cost of the Hepatitis B vaccine, compared to all other EPI vaccines has brought in the notion of 'vaccine security'. Introduction of the HB vaccine also has implications for training of staff, change of immunisation forms, advocacy and communication campaigns. The WHO is advocating inclusion of quadrivalent vaccines (DPT-HB) in the UIP to reduce number of injections per visit, needles and syringes and storage space; however, the quadrivalent vaccine implies pushing up the costs astronomically (http://www.who.int/vaccines, 2004 and http://www.who.int/emc, 2004).

In the overall epidemiology of chronic liver diseases in India, the contribution of Hepatitis B *vis-a-vis* other dominant causes such as malnutrition and alcoholism is yet to be clearly established. Rigorous implementation of the practice of universal precautions for infection control in medical practice and limiting sexual transmission are common measures for minimising spread of both HIV/AIDS and Hepatitis B with scope for convergence of the two programmes. Interventions in social and professional processes may require much less financial inputs, but far more intense human interaction to change attitudes and attain sustainable results. The stand-alone strategy of universal immunisation will have limited impact on the overall prevalence of Hepatitis B and the synchronisation with the DPT schedule will have negative implications for prevention of chronic complications as well. There is need for both research and debate and the announcement of the policy should not forestall either of these.

III. The Case of the Oral Polio Vaccine

The 1983 conference in Bellagio, Italy, put forward the notion of global polio eradication as a goal for the Expanded Programme of Immunisation (EPI) (John, 1996). In 1984, Rotary International constituted a consultative committee to consider the potential of a global effort against poliomyelitis. Based on the committee's report, Rotary International declared the goal of poliomyelitis eradication by 2005. In 1985, the Pan American Health Organization (PAHO) adopted a resolution to eradicate polio from the Western Hemisphere by 1990. The World Health Assembly of 1988 adopted the resolution for global eradication of polio by 2000.

It is unfortunate that 'eradication' and 'elimination' are used interchangeably. The Dahlem Workshop on the Eradication of Infectious Diseases held in 1997 defined 'eradication' as 'permanent reduction to zero of the worldwide incidence of infection caused by a specific agent as a result of deliberate efforts; intervention measures are no longer needed' (Dowdle, 1998). The Global Commission for the Certification of the Eradication of Poliomyelitis defined eradication as the absence of circulation of all indigenous wild polioviruses for at least a three-year period during which surveillance activities had been maintained at the levels of performance needed for certification (WHO, 1998). 'Elimination of Infections' was defined by the Dahlem Workshop as '...Reduction to zero of the worldwide incidence of infection caused by a specific agent in a defined geographical area as a result of deliberate efforts; continued measurements to prevent re-establishment of transmission are required. Example: measles and poliomyelitis' (Dowdle, 1998).

Considering the Indian scenario, the first tenet of the four principal strategies of eradication—strengthening the ongoing routine immunisation—was never followed. On the contrary, routine coverage weakened following the Pulse Polio Immunisation (PPI) strategy. Paediatricians have reported re-emergence of some of the vaccine preventable diseases like tuberculous meningitis and diphtheria that had almost disappeared in the last one decade. The Planning Commission, drawing upon the data from the National Family Health Survey, mentions the adverse impact of PPI on routine immunization programmes (Planning Commission, Tenth Plan, undated).

Large variation has been reported in routine immunisation coverage across Indian states—from 97 per cent in Kerala to 21 per cent in Bihar (CDC, 2003). A coverage evaluation by the UNICEF reported consistently low routine (and PPI) coverage in these states and some others like Rajasthan. In Bihar, the OPV3 ranged from 21-25 per cent in the last few years. In 2002 it was 35 per cent in Rajasthan and 41 per cent in UP in 2001-02. Over-emphasis on PPI rounds and other supplemental rounds were identified as causes of 'fatigue' thereby leaving vast pools of unimmunised children. Up to 15 per cent of children were missed during mop-up rounds. "It is essential that routine immunization coverage in infants in all states be maintained well above 85-90 per cent (Thacker, 2004)." Contrary to popular belief, majority of the children who were afflicted by paralytic poliomyelitis due to wild poliovirus in both the confirmed and compatible category had received more than 3 doses of OPV (Satyamala et al, 2005).

In the context of India both immune deficiency and intramuscular injections could be considered major factors for increasing the risk of paralysis. A retrospective, population-based study on paralytic poliomyelitis in rural Haryana showed that 60 per cent of children developed paralysis soon after they were given an intramuscular injection (Varghese et al, 1997). In the post-GPEI period in India too provocative paralysis due to intramuscular injections has been indicted as an important cause of paralysis. A recently published case-control study on the outbreak of poliomyelitis in UP (1999-2000) has confirmed that history of an injection was significantly associated with the risk of paralysis (adjusted odds ratio = 3.9; 95 per cent CI: 1.8-12.5) (Kohler et al, 2003). The injections had been given 30 days before the onset of paralysis. However, none of the IEC (Information, Education, Communication) material, prepared by the UNICEF, and used in the Pulse Polio campaign breathes a word about this key risk factor. Not including such contraindication in the publicity materials tantamount to unethical practice which would not be allowed to any pharmaceutical company for its products.

There is considerable confusion in perceptions about the journey ahead. A campaign on the eve of the SNID on 9th January, 2005, featuring the Union Health and Family Welfare Minister and also the Minister of State was misleadingly captioned 'Freedom From Polio Within Six Months' (*Times of India*, January 8, 2005)! In the 'post-eradication strategy' the introduction of the Injectable Polio Vaccine (IPV) is being actively propagated (Mathew et al, 2002; Kalra et al, 2002). The Tenth Plan document also hails IPV as a 'superior' vaccine within the eradication initiative and as part of routine immunisation programme. John (2003) explored the issue in great detail. Projecting the certification of 'eradication' of wild viruses in 2006, after achieving 'elimination of transmission' in 2003, he advised the introduction of IPV in the same year. While OPV (and VAPP) will continue for another three years, till 2009, 'true eradication' can be certified only in 2012. The IPV discontinuation will finally be achieved in 2015; all milestones will be correspondingly delayed if 'elimination' is delayed, which is clearly the case. Further, John also recommended that a quadrivalent DPT-IPV be introduced into the routine immunisation programme. With Hepatitis B also being included in the National Immunisation Schedule (in a phased manner), is the stage being set for a pentavalent vaccine? If IPV is introduced, the country will face a cost burden that would be far higher than the OPV campaign. Price war and murky deals witnessed with the Hepatitis B vaccine is unavoidable

Discussion

Child immunisation has been hailed as one of the most cost-effective health interventions (World Bank, 1993). Global Alliance for Vaccines and Immunisation (GAVI) is under contract with several large multi-national corporations that manufacture and market vaccines. GAVI resisted pressure from countries with generic-drug industries including India to transfer patented vaccine technologies to manufacturers in poorer countries (Madhavi, 2003). In an uncanny similarity with the Pulse Polio Programme, UNICEF (with strong links with multi-national corporations) has emerged as the procurement agency for the HB vaccine in the UIP. GAVI recognises that data on magnitude of the disease burden and programme conditions are weak in developing countries; nevertheless, it pushes Hepatitis B vaccination through loans for limited periods.

Vaccines alone have limited role in control of diseases. Its relevance in the total package of control measures need to be articulated clearly. Otherwise, despite immense commitment of resources, favourable outcomes will continue to elude us. With renewed emphasis on the UIP both in the NRHM and in the context of the inability to eradicate polio as per earlier schedules, immunisation has been hailed as the 'one' solution to a range of infections in recent catch-up campaigns. Immunisation is being oversold ignoring the epidemiological complexities of diseases and is being picked up as a soft option coupled with the lack of local thinking and global public health prescriptions. Caution needs to be sounded regarding this 'universal' solution and realistic expectations need to be kept in mind, particularly since these are extremely cost and human resource intensive operations.

REFERENCES

1. Aggarwal R. and Ghoshal U.C., 'Hepatitis B Vaccination Policy for India: Is selective vaccination an option?' *Indian Journal of Gastroenterology,* 23 (1), 2-4, 2004.
2. CDC-Progress towards polio eradication, *MMWR* 2003; 52: 172-175, India 2002.
3. Damme V. P., 'Viral Hepatitis Fact Sheet 1 January', *Fact Sheet* VHPB/1996/1.
4. Dasgupta R., 'Universalising the Hepatitis B Vaccine in India; Pitfalls in Policy and Practice', *Journal of Health and Development,* Vol. 1, Nos. 2&3, 2005.
5. Dasgupta R., Priya R., 'The Sustainability of Hepatitis B Immunisation within the Universal Immunisation Programme in India', *Health Policy and Planning,* 17(1):99-105, 2002.
6. Dowdle W. R., 'The Principles of Disease Elimination and Eradication', in Global Disease Elimination and Eradication as Public Health Strategies, *Bulletin of the World Health Organization* 76 (2): 22-25, 1998.
7. Government of India, http://mohfw.nic.in/IME-revised.pdf. visited on 11.01.2005, 2004.
8. Grundy E., 'Commentary: The McKeown Debate—Time for Burial', *International Journal of Epidemiology,* 34: 529-533, 2005.
9. http://www.childliverdisease.org/education/HepBvaccampaign, accessed on 09.09.2005.

10. *http://www.who.int/emc- documents/hepatitis/docs/whocdscsrlyo20022/treatment/hepatitis_immunization.html.* (2004). Introducing hepatitis B vaccine into national immunization services.
11. *http://www.who.int/vaccines-diseases/diseases/hepatitis_b.shtml.*(2004). Hepatitis B Vaccine, Public Health Strategies, 2004.
12. Hyams, K.C., 'Risks of Chronicity Following Acute Hepatitis B Virus Infection: A Review', *Clin Infect Dis.*, 20:992-1000, 2005.
13. John, T. J., 'Can We Eradicate Poliomyelitis?' In, Sachdev H. P. S and Choudhury P (eds), *Frontiers in Paediatrics,* pp. 76-90, Jaypee Brothers Medical Publishers (P) Ltd, New Delhi, 1996.
14. John T.J., 'Polio Eradication in India: What is the Future?' *Indian Paediatrics,* 2003; 455-462.
15. Kalra K.K., Mittal S.K., 'Polio-Free India: Can we make the dream come true?' *Paediatrics Today.*5(6): 339-346, 2002.
16. Kohler K.A., Hlady W.G., Banerji K., Sutter R.W., 'Outbreak of Poliomyelitis Due to Type 3 Poliovirus, Northern India, 1999-2000: Injections a Major Contributing Factor', *International Journal of Epidemiology.* 32:272-277, 2003.
17. Lai C.L., Ratziu V., Yuen M., Poynard T., 'Viral Hepatitis B', *Lancet,* 362: 2089-94, 2003.
18. Madhavi Y., 'Manufacture of Consent? Hepatitis B vaccination', *Economic and Political Weekly,* June 14, 2003.
19. Mathew J. L., Gera T., Mittal S.K., 'Eradication of Poliomyelitis in India – Future Perspectives', *Paediatrics* 3(10):647- 660, 2002.
20. McKeown T., Brown R.G. and Record R.G., An Interpretation of the Modern Rise of Population in Europe, 1992.
21. Mohandas K.M., 'Epidemiology of HBV-associated Hepatocellular Carcinoma in India', *Indian Journal of Gastroenterology,* 19 (Supplement 3): December 2000.
22. Phadke A. and Kale A, 'Some Critical Issues in the Epidemiology of Hepatitis B in India', *Indian Journal of Gastroenterology,* 19 (Supplement 3): December 2000.
23. Planning Commission, Tenth Five-Year Plan (2002-2007), Volume II, Sectoral Policies and Programmes, Family Welfare, Government of India, New Delhi, undated.
24. Planning Commission, Tenth Five-Year Plan (2002-2007), Volume II, Sectoral Policies and Programmes, Family Welfare, Government of India, New Delhi, undated.
25. Sahni M., Jindal K., Abraham N., Aruldas K., Puliyel J., 'Hepatitis B Immunization: Cost Calculation in a Community-Based Study in India', *Indian Journal of Gastroenterology,* 23 (1), 16-18, 2004.
26. Sathyamala C., Mittal O., Dasgupta R., Priya R., 'Polio Eradication Initiative in India', *International Journal of Health Services,* 35(2): 361-383, 2005.
27. Thacker N., Shendurnikar N., 'Current status of polio eradication and future prospects', *Indian Journal of Paediatrics,* 71:241-245, 2004.
28. 'Prime Minister Vajpayee Launches New Initiative to Vaccinate Children Against Hepatitis B', June 10, 2002, *The Hindu*.
29. Thyagarajan, S.P., 'Prevalence of Hepatitis B Virus Infection in General Population of India', *Indian Journal of Gastroenterology,* 19 (Supplement 3): December.
30. DAVP Advertisement No. 2004/574, January 8, 2005, *Times of India.*

31. 'Hepatitis B Threat Eclipses AIDS', September 5, 2005, *Times of India.*
32. Varghese M., Qadeer I., Mohan D., 'Paralytic Poliomyelitis in a Rural Area in North India', *The National Medical Journal of India,* 10 (1): 8-10, 1997.
33. WHO, Report of the Second Meeting of the Global Commission for the Certification of the Eradication of Poliomyelitis. http://www.who.int. Geneva 1 May, 1997; pp 2 and 8, 1998.
34. World Health Organisation, WHO Expanded Programme on Immunisation, Hepatitis B Control Through Immunisation, Global Programme for Vaccines and Immunisation Sub-Committee Meeting of the Scientific Advisory Group of Experts, Geneva, 12th–16th June 1995.
35. World Bank, World Development Report 1993, Investing in Health, Oxford University Press, 1993, Oxford.
36. www.vaccinealliance.org: Vaccines are Cost-Effective: A Summary of Recent Research. Health, Immunisation and Economic Growth, Research Briefing 2, www.vaccinealliance.org, GAVI.

SECTION II

Financing of Healthcare Services

4

Changing Patterns in Public Expenditure on Reproductive and Child Health Services in India

T R Dilip

Introduction

Currently the public of reproductive and child healthcare services are tax financed and delivered through a large network of over 1.4 lakh subcentres and over 50,000 PHCs/dispensaries and other secondary care institutions spread across the country. There have been profound changes in India's health and population policies since the year 2000. It started with the National Population Policy (NPP) 2000, which gave an increased emphasis on delivery of RCH services which, in addition to family planning, includes antenatal and postnatal care, childbirth assistance, child healthcare, and treatment of reproductive tract infections (GoI 2000). The NPP had taken a serious note on financial deficiency in public provision of contraceptive services (Rs 150 crores), health infrastructure (Rs 6400 crores), trained manpower (Rs 2300 crores) and training (Rs 10 crores). But the deficit mentioned above is more than the total public expenditure on health and is prepared on assumption that all will prefer the public sector for all these types of services. Further 50 per cent of budget allocation of Department of Family Welfare, Ministry of Health and Family Welfare is for salaries and maintenance of infrastructure in states and Union Territories, while only the remaining 50 per cent is for 'plan activities' including purchase of equipments (GoI 2000). However, this policy was largely silent on financing strategies for improvement in public spending including that for RCH services. But the whole initiative to collaborate with voluntary organisations, NGOs and industry may be seen as an option for improving the financial resources available for RCH care in future.

After that the National Health Policy 2002 was formulated, which envisaged a key role for the Central Government in designing and supporting health programmes in the country with the active participation of the state government. RCH activities were in the forefront on NHP agenda which had made a commitment towards eradication of polio and reduction in levels of Infant Mortality and Maternal mortality (GoI 2002). Financing targets in NHP 2002 are very specific as: (1) raising government expenditure on health from present level of 0.9 per cent to two per cent by the year 2010; (2) state governments to increase allocations to health to seven per cent of budget by 2005 and eight per cent by 2010; (3) Central Government contribution to increase from 15 per cent to 25 per cent; and (4) pattern of public investment in primary, secondary and tertiary sectors to be 55, 35 and 10 per cent respectively. Therefore, the condition in general can be expected to be favourable for augmenting public spending on health, including RCH services.

Since then we have the National Common Minimum Programme formulated in the year 2004 where one agenda is to step up the public expenditure on health to two to three per cent of GDP with focus on primary care. The National Rural Health Mission (NRHM), an outcome of commitments made in NCMP in order to address this issue of augmenting health infrastructure and promoting health seeking behaviour through higher access. Hence at the policy level the conditions are favourable for an increase in public spending, and there is a need to find out where is the financial resources are coming from and where does it go. This paper examines the same in the case of reproductive and child health services.

Public Expenditure on Healthcare Services

The public expenditure on health is far from adequate and remains at a stagnant level of around 0.9 per cent of GDP for the last one decade. Critics associate the deterioration in public health system also to falling levels of public health investment and the declining public health expenditure (Duggal 2005). Public expenditure on health accounts for nearly 22 per cent of the total health expenditure in India (NCMH 2005). NCMH report further point out that salaries and wages account for 70 per cent of health budget, while only 12 per cent is drugs medicines, supplies and consumables, eight per cent for purchase of machinery and equipment, five per cent on maintenance of buildings, equipments etc and remaining five per cent on other routine expenditures. Though health is a state subject the state governments too have limited resources to invest in healthcare including RCH care services. Available evidence on health spending by state governments suggests allocation to health sector in the total budget to be declining between 1985-86 and 1998-1999 (Selvaraj and Annegeri 2000). This trend is likely to continue since 2000 due to the ongoing fiscal reform process across states.

Demand for RCH Services in India

As known there is a huge demand for RCH services in India. This is despite of the fact that a sizeable proportion of the country population is not accessing RCH services (Table 1). Apart from the above observation there are large scale inequalities in assessing these services between lower and higher standards of living sub groups. Demand for RCH services is likely to increase sharply when these subgroups of population becomes closer to heath care system resulting in utilization of these services. One again has to note that most of the indicators mentioned below are outside the risk/resource

Table 1: Gaps in Utilization of RCH Services in India

Indicator	%
Pregnant women with no ANC check-up	34.0
Pregnant women without TT injection	24.1
Pregnant women not receiving IFA tablet/syrup	42.4
Non-institutional deliveries	66.4
Births not attended by medical professionals	57.4
Women not receiving post-partum check-up	73.5
Current contraceptive use (women 15-44 years)	48.2
Children fully immunized	42.0
Children not receiving Vitamin A supplementation	29.7

Source: IIPS and ORC Macro (2002).

pooling strategy which is often proposed as one of the alternatives to finance healthcare services in India. In this regard provision of these services through public outlets through improved resource allocation seems to be the main option for ensuring access to safe RCH services for subgroups of population who are yet to get acquainted with these types of services. Present evidence shows Reproductive and Child Health is grossly underfunded and the estimated deficit is to the tune of 4267 crore rupees for the year 2001-02 (NCMH 2005). This accounts for 77 per cent of the estimated under-funding in national health programmes for the year.

Expenditure on RCH Services

This overall picture in public spending on health is to be noted while analysing the expenditure on RCH services, which is a major component within India's health budget. Results from Rajasthan indicate that public sector accounts for 28 per cent and 21 per cent of total health spending and total spending on RCH care, respectively (IIHMR et al, 2000). For Andhra Pradesh the expenditure on the same was 27 per cent and 29 per cent, respectively (George and Patnaik, 2005). Disaggregate data on financing of RCH services is limited when compared to data on health financing in India. In addition the ability to analyse government expenditure on reproductive health and to track them over time is reported to be limited in India as elsewhere in the developing countries (Berman, 2004). The government expenditure on RCH services can be traced from the budget documents of Ministry of Health and Family Welfare and the budgets of State Department of Health in each state and Union Territories with legislature. But private expenditure on reproductive and child health services, mainly the out-of-pocket expenditure by households is largely unexplored due to unavailability of data. Indirect estimates based on data extrapolated using small-scale studies given in the NCMH report show that 9.1 per cent of the total household out-of-pocket expenditure on health is for delivery care, ante/post-natal care, immunization and contraception. However, the NCMH (2005) does not provide disaggregated data for public expenditure on RCH services.

In this background, the present analysis focuses on the nature of changes in public spending on RCH services ever since the formulation of National Population Policy in 2000 and National

Health Policy in the year 2002. As known, there has been a change in investment pattern with the launch of the National Rural Health Mission in the year 2005. However, financial data on actual expenditure is not available for period beyond 2003-04 but the analysis is mainly based on limited data on 'revised estimates' for the year 2004-05 and 'budget estimates' for the year 2005-06.

Central Government Expenditure

Since the Central Government grants constitute most of public spending on family welfare activities in states (Selvaraju and Annegeri, 2000), analysis of Central Government expenditure provides valuable insights into source and use of funds for family welfare services through the public sector in India. Health expenditure by the Central Government is 4311 crore rupees for the year 2004-05 (Table 2). The allocation is expected to nearly double by the year 2006-07. There is a substantial level of increase in health expenditure between these periods in nominal terms. Health expenditure as a percentage of total Central Government expenditure increases from 0.31 per cent in 1999-2000 to 0.4 per cent in the year 2003-04, which is likely to touch 0.46 per cent by the year 2006-07. However there was a remarkable increase in expenditure on family welfare especially after the release of NHP in the year 2002. One can

Table 2: Trends in Health Expenditure by Central Government

(actual expenditure in crores of rupees)

	(a) Exp. on Medical and Public Health	(b) Exp. on Family Welfare	(c) Total Health Expenditure@ (a+b)	(d) Total Expenditure# Health exp.	as % total exp. Family Welfare exp.	as % of health exp.
1999-2000	1637	521	2158	704639	0.31	24.2
2000-2001	1811	661	2472	665347	0.37	26.7
2001-2002	2062	765	2827	767216	0.37	27.1
2002-2003	2231	797	3028	815987	0.37	26.3
2003-2004	2495	1266	3761	937780	0.40	33.7
2004-2005	2915	1397	4311	1105602	0.39	32.4
2005-2006[1] (RE)	3288	2964	6252	1634820	0.38	47.4
2006-2007[2] (BE)	4109	4019	8128	1752018	0.46	49.4

@ expenditure under the major heads '2210', '2211' and '4210'.
# Total consolidated fund of India disbursements.
[1] Revised estimate; [2] Budget estimate.
Source: Compiled from Annual Financial Statement for respective years.

see family welfare expenditure as a percentage of total expenditure to increase from 24 in 1999-2000 to 49 by the year 2006-07. All this indicate that enhancement observed in health sector allocation by the Centre is mainly due to the higher importance given to family welfare activities in their health budget.

State Government Expenditure

The reverse scenario was observed in the case of state government's expenditure on medical and public health and family welfare services. Health expenditure as a percentage of total expenditure has declined from 4.8 in 1999-2000 to 2.9 in 2003-04. There was no notable hike in allocation for family welfare/RCH activities by the states. Here it is to be cited that a sizeable share of the health expenditure shown in Table 3 is using funds received as a part of grant in aid from the Central Government. Hence in total one can assume that there is a severe decline in health spending by state governments since the 2000s. It looks like state governments are not in a position to keep pace with the policy changes of the Central Government due to fiscal constraints.

Table 3: Trends in Health Expenditure by State Governments

(actual expenditure in crores of rupees)

	(a) Exp. on Medical and Public Health	(b) Exp. on Family Welfare	(c) Total Health Expenditure@ (a+b)	(d) Total Expenditure#	as % total Health exp.	as % of health exp. Family Welfare exp.
1999-2000	12917	2140	15058	313889	4.8	14.2
2000-2001	13742	2398	16140	347198	4.6	14.9
2001-2002	14114	2513	16627	377312	4.4	15.1
2002-2003	14700	2393	17094	420462	4.1	14.0
2003-2004	15735	2500	18235	638902	2.9	13.7
2004-2005[1] (RE)	18311	3154	21465	662967	3.2	14.7
2005-2006[2] (BE)	20967	3369	24336	624060	3.9	13.8

@ expenditure under the major heads '2210', '2211', '4210' and '4211'.

Includes total revenue expenditure, capital disbursement, discharge of internal debt, repayments of loans to the Centre and loans and advances by the state government.

[1] Revised estimate; [2] Budget estimate.

Source: Compiled from RBI annual publication titled 'State Finances: A Study of Budgets for Respective Years.

Reproductive and Child Health Expenditure by Central Government

In Table 4 we analyze expenditure on Reproductive and Child Health Services incurred by the Central Government by their original source of funds. This expenditure is incurred in two ways: (1) Through the annual budget of Ministry of Health and Family Welfare (MOHFW), and (2) Grant-in-aid from MOHFW Budget to State/ Union Territories for carrying out health activities. As is known, the Central Government utilizes funds received in the form of External Assistance Component (External Support) for financing healthcare activities. This component is separated to get the expenditure incurred by funds for healthcare from the Central Government revenue.

The Central Government expenditure on family welfare component including expenditure by the Ministry of Health and Family Welfare and Grant-in-aid to States/UTs increased from 3673 crore rupees in 2000-01 to 5191 crore rupees by 2003-04. Nearly 72 per cent of these funds are from Central Government revenue and rest is external aid component. A marginal decline in external support component was noted during these four years. These is a gradual rise in funds from own revenue out of total funds disbursed by the central government from 72 per cent in 2000-01 to 76 per cent in 2003-04.

The state government incurs health expenditure in two ways: (1) Through the state government funds and (2) Grant-in-aid from Central Government (which includes external support component also). Only a few of the states receive direct funding from abroad and their contribution is low and one has to analyze all state government budgets to separate this out. Since centrally sponsored schemes account for a major chunk of the state government expenditure on RCH/Family Welfare services (Shown in Table 3), an overview on their use of funds could be obtained from the Central Government budget itself.

Source of Funds for Central and State Government Expenditure on RCH Services

Source of funds for RCH services is presented in Table 5. Out of the total expenditure by Central and state governments on RCH services, during this period one can find that Central Government

Table 4: Reproductive and Child Health Expenditure by MOHFW by Source of Funds

(actual expenditure in crores of rupees)

	Exp incurred by MOHFW			Grant-in-aid by MOHFW to States & UTs			Total Exp. by MOHFW	% Exp. by MOHFW from own funds
	Budget support (1)	External support$ (2)	Total (3) = (1)+(2)	Budget support (4)	External support (5)	Total (6)=(4)+(5)	(7)=(3)+(5)	((1)+(4))/(7))*100
2000-01	661	570	1232	1990	452	2442	3673	72.2
2001-02	765	589	1354	2242	498	2739	4093	73.5
2002-03	797	675	1472	2646	540	3186	4658	73.9
2003-04	1266	761	2027	2694	470	3165	5191	76.3
2004-05 (RE)	1458	973	2431	2621	712	3332	5763	70.8
2005-06 (BE)	2272	1316	3588	2880	655	3535	7122	72.3

$ This includes aid materials and equipments under the major head 3606

Source: Compiled from Demand for Grants, Ministry of Health and Family Welfare for respective years.

funds for RCH services have increased by 49 per cent while it is only 20 per cent in the case of external assistance.

Table 5: Source of Funds for Public Expenditure on RCH Services

	Source of funds			Percentage of funds from		
	Central Govt.	External Support	Total	Central Govt	External Support	Total
2000-01	265088	102217	367305	72.2	27.8	100.0
2001-02	300618	108647	409265	73.5	26.5	100.0
2002-03	344315	121521	465836	73.9	26.1	100.0
2003-04	396060	123080	519140	76.3	23.7	100.0
Growth rate 2000-01 to 2003-04 (%)	49.4	20.4	41.3			

Whatever rise in public expenditure on RCH services observed during the above period is mainly due to the Central Government's contribution.

Utilization of Funds Available for RCH

Table 6 gives information expenditure on RCH services by various functions. Nearly 76 per cent of expenditure is under the head Reproductive and Child Health Project. Services and supplies account for 12.2 per cent. Funds allocated for functions like training, mass education and research and evaluation were relatively very low.

At the aggregate level one can find that the overall increase in public expenditure on RCH is mainly due to increased allocation for the RCH project. Here the major components in the RCH project are the National Immunisation Programme and polio eradication.

Table 7 shows how the grant-in-aid from Central Government to states and union territories for family welfare activities is getting used. State governments utilize more than 50 per cent of these grants for strengthening rural family welfare services. Expenditure on rural family welfare services increased from 41 per cent in 2000-01 to 54 per cent by the year 2003-04. Government spending on maternal and child health/RCH project has also increased from 20 per cent to 30 per cent during the above period.

Since the figures are from budgets of MOHFW, any expenditure on family welfare by state government other than grant-in-aid from Central Government is not accounted in here.

Table 6: Percentage Distribution of RCH Expenditure by Ministry of Health and Family Welfare by Functions

Functions	Percentage of expenditure in					
	2000-01	2001-02	2002-03	2003-04	2004-05	2005-06
Direction and Administration	1.0	0.9	0.8	0.5	0.5	0.4
Training	1.5	1.5	1.5	1.2	1.2	0.9
Research and Evaluation	1.8	2.0	2.1	2.0	1.7	1.2
Rural Family Welfare Services	0.2	0.2	0.2	0.2	0.1	1.7
Urban Family Welfare Services	0.1	0.1	0.0	0.0	0.0	0.0
Reproductive and Child Health Project	63.3	57.7	61.2	61.1	60.2	75.9
Compensation	0.0	0.0	0.0	0.0	0.0	0.0
Mass education	1.7	2.6	3.9	0.0	6.9	3.5
Selected Area Programmes	10.1	7.0	2.5	1.7	1.7	1.5
Services and supplies	16.3	17.0	20.1	16.2	14.9	12.2
Other expenditure	3.8	10.9	7.6	17.2	12.7	2.7
Total	100.0	100.0	100.0	100.0	100.0	100.0
Total expenditure (in crores of Rupees)	1193	1296	1348	1768	2300	3458

Source: # Compiled from Demand for Grants, Ministry of Health and Family Welfare for respective years.
Figures for the 2004-05 are revised estimates and for 2005-06 are budget estimates.

Table 7: Utilization of Grant-in-aid for Family Welfare Activities from Central Government by State/UT Governments by Functions

Functions	Percentage of expenditure in					
	2000-01	2001-02	2002-03	2003-04	2004-05	2005-06
Urban Family Welfare Services	4.4	4.8	3.2	3.7	3.6	3.7
Maternity and Child Health/RCH project	20.2	17.6	16.6	19.2	25.8	30.4
Transport	3.2	2.5	3.5	2.5	1.5	0.0
Compensation	4.8	4.5	4.7	6.3	5.9	0.0
Other services and supplies	4.1	4.4	4.9	4.6	2.8	4.8
Mass education	0.4	0.0	0.0	0.0	0.0	0.0
Training	2.3	2.9	2.6	2.9	2.7	2.8
Selected Area Projects	3.3	3.5	0.8	0.1	0.0	0.0
Direction and Administration	4.3	3.9	5.7	6.6	6.1	7.1
Rural Family Welfare services	40.7	41.9	57.9	54.1	51.6	51.2
Other grants	12.3	13.9	0.0	0.0	0.0	0.0
Total	100	100	100	100	100	100
Total Grant-in-aid (in crores of Rupees)	2442	2739	3186	3165	3332	3535

Source: # Compiled from Demand for Grants, Ministry of Health and Family Welfare for respective years.
Figures for the 2004-05 are revised estimates and for 2005-06 are budget estimates.

The aggregate data on public spending on RCH services (Central + State government) is presented in Table 8. This also shows that priority for the expenditure head 'Maternal and Child Health/RCH Project' has increased over time. More than 50 per cent of the funds are allocated under this head, where immunization is the major component. Notable improvement in expenditure on rural family welfare services was also not observed during this period. Expenditure on functions like training, research and evaluation services and supplies has declined. A significant increase in expenditure under the head mass education was observed.

Conclusion

There has been a sizeable improvement in public expenditure on Reproductive and Child Health Services especially with the beginning of the National Rural Health Mission initiative. This has helped in bridging the gap quantum of under-spending in the RCH services mentioned in the National Population Policy 2000 to a certain extent. However, the effort to improve expenditure on health including RCH services has primarily come from the Central Government. The state governments which were in the midst of fiscal crisis during their efforts to reduce expenditure were not found to be giving due attention to health sector. Again the health and population policy changes have been confined to the Central Government and necessary alteration are yet to take place at the state level in financing of health services. Even after 50 years of implementation of family planning/welfare programme, it continues to be a centrally sponsored one. Component-wise imbalances in funds allocated for RCH services were noticed. Components like urban family welfare services, training and research and evaluation require more attention. Similarly major share of expenditure under the RCH project, which has the largest share in family welfare budget, is for strengthening the National Immunisation Programme. Intensive analysis is necessary at regular intervals to ascertain the capacity of financing strategies in filling the gaps in access to RCH services across India.

Table 8: Utilization of Funds Allocated for Family Welfare Activities by Central and State Governments

Functions	Percentage of expenditure in					
	2000-01	2001-02	2002-03	2003-04	2004-05	2005-06
Direction and Administration	5.4	4.7	6.7	6.1	4.7	3.8
Training	2.1	2.4	2.3	2.3	2.1	1.9
Research and Evaluation	0.6	0.7	0.6	0.7	0.7	0.6
Rural Family Welfare Services	27.4	23.5	40.8	34.7	30.6	26.7
Urban Family Welfare services	3.0	3.3	2.3	2.4	2.1	1.9
Maternal and Child Health/RCH Project	34.3	30.5	29.8	34.2	39.8	52.9
Compensation	3.3	3.0	3.3	4.0	3.5	0.0
Mass education	0.8	0.8	1.1	0.0	2.8	1.7
Selected Area Programmes	5.5	4.6	1.3	0.7	0.7	0.7
Services and supplies	8.1	8.4	9.4	8.7	7.7	8.5
Other expenditure	9.5	12.9	2.3	6.2	5.2	1.4
Total	100	100	100	100	100	100
Total RCH expenditure (in Rupees crores)#	3634	4035	4534	4933	5632	6992

Source: # Compiled from Demand for Grants, Ministry of Health and Family Welfare for respective years.
Figures for the 2004-05 are revised estimates and for 2005-06 are budget estimates.

REFERENCES

1. Berman P., 'Financing and payment reforms relevant to RCH programmes: Global trends and recent experience in India', Paper prepared for Technical Consultation on Health Sector Reform and Reproductive Health: Developing the Evidence Base, Geneva, 30th November- 2nd December 2004.
2. Duggal R., 'Public Health Expenditure, Investment and Financing under the Shadow of a Growing Private Sector' in Ganguly et al ed, *Review of Healthcare in India*, Centre for Enquiry into Health and Allied Themes, Mumbai, 2005.
3. George C.K. and Patnaik G.S., 'Andhra Pradesh State Health Accounts 2001-02', Institute of Health Systems, Hyderabad, 2004.
4. Government of India, 'National Population Policy 2000', Department of Family Welfare, Ministry of Health and Family Welfare, Government of India, New Delhi, 2002.
5. Government of India, 'National Health Policy 2002', Department of Health, Ministry of Health and Family Welfare, Government of India, New Delhi, 2002.
6. Government of India, 'National Rural Health Mission: Mission Document', Ministry of Health and Family Welfare, Government of India, New Delhi, 2005.
7. Government of India, Demand for Grants for Ministry of Health and Family Welfare, respective years.
8. International Institute for Population Sciences (IIPS) and ORC Macro, National Family Health Survey (NFHS-2), 1998-99, IIPS, Mumbai, 2000.
9. Indian Institute of Health Management and Futures Group International 'Reproductive and Child Healthcare in Rajasthan', IIHMR, Jaipur, 2000.
10. National Commission on Macro Economics and Health, 'Financing and Delivery of Healthcare Services in India', Ministry of Health and Family Welfare, Government of India, New Delhi, 2005.
11. Reserve Bank of India, 'State Finances Study of Budgets', respective years.
12. Selvaraj V. and Annegeri V., 'Trends in Public Spending on Health in India', New Delhi: National Institute of Public Finance and Policy (Unpublished research document, 2000).

5

Financing Health – Some Issues and Concerns for Mother and Child

Sanghmitra S Acharya

Background

Provision of universal and comprehensive healthcare is the central concern of the governments of developing countries where the healthcare coverage continues to be limited. The decades of 1970s and 1980s experienced expansion of the public health sector in the developing countries. The WHO resolution in the International Conference on Primary Healthcare at Alma Ata in 1978 called for the government health policies to ensure provisioning of healthcare to all, specially the under-privileged. As a result, A 'Primary Healthcare Model' was advocated by the WHO which emphasized the need to build and sustain national health systems to meet the needs of all, particularly the vulnerable populations. The goal of 'Health for All by 2000' was set. WHO recommended an outlay of five per cent of the GDP for which the state was expected to raise additional resources. The additional finance was to be borne by the public sector. However, the goal of providing universal healthcare for the people is still a distant dream. A vast majority of population still lack access to basic curative and preventive healthcare systems.

During the late 1960s and 1970s developing countries were experiencing global recession, worsening terms of trade and high burden of international debt. The deepening economic recession during the 1970s started showing an impact on the health financing policies of the developing countries. The economic recession in the developed countries, rise in the oil prices, and the fall in the prices of the raw materials which constituted the main exports from developing countries compounded their problem and reflected on their economic dependence on the developed countries. They were left with little option in accepting the structural adjustment programmes of the World Bank to salvage their economies. Severe curtailment of public expenditure for social sector and limiting state intervention called for a rethink on financing and delivering healthcare especially to the vulnerable populations. Public sector has been historically responsible for meeting the health needs of the weaker sections of the society both in developed and developing countries.

Public financing of health services expanded considerably to provide near-universal coverage to the people in the developed countries during the 1960s and the 1970s. However, the onset of recession, slowing down of economic growth, and advent of costly medical technologies and the growing proportion of the aged population set the limit for expansion of public expenditure. Regulation of health expenditure for cost containment and greater use of private alternatives to fund healthcare became important concerns. This change in public sector expenditure on health services opened up the issue of alternative methods and sources of financing healthcare. Since the mid-1980s the issue of alternative methods of financing healthcare in the developing countries has been a major concern. Governments were expected to directly finance or subsidise healthcare. Alternatives proposed for the developing countries included greater role for private sector, user-fee for government services, expanding private insurance schemes and developing schemes for community financing.

The under-privileged populations in the developing countries are yet to be ensured basic minimum healthcare. Despite the increase in public financing of health services and expansion of health facilities and medical care in the government sector, access continues to be unsatisfactory. In developing countries like India, the vast burden of healthcare expenses are borne by individual households, particularly the poor, due to limited government services and a rapidly growing 'for-profit' private sector in curative care. This reflects on the issue whether the alternatives are in consonance with the ideal of equitable, universal access to healthcare goal.

Health Sector Planning and Mother and Child Health

The present health system in India, like most other countries with a colonial past, has its origin in the colonial administration. The system overlooked the poor and the rural masses. They were not covered by the official health programmes. This pattern is evident even today in more than one way. The location of mother and child in the health sector has been largely determined by two factors responsible for shaping the population policy of India—

1. Population growth as one of the determinants of poverty and therefore need to check it for national development.
2. Benefits accruing to women's health through acceptance of contraception and limiting the family size.

The thrust given to population control to usher in 'better standards of living' and 'good health for women' actually turned out to be a reiteration of women as agents of procreation than anything else. So much so that the Health Survey and Development Committee, better known as Bhore Committee (Bhore et al 1946), was established towards the end of the British rule in 1943 to assess the provisioning of health services in the country. Mother and child health formed a separate segment in the larger health framework. It was endorsed in the Alma Ata conference where 'Mother and Child Health' (MCH) was the approach to health for all through primary healthcare. This was broadened to 'Child Survival and Safe Motherhood' (CSSM) during the late 1980s and through the 1990s, and then to 'reproductive health' and 'Reproductive and Child Health' (RCH) after the International Conference on Population and Development (ICPD) held in Cairo in 1994. This added the dimension of responsible parenthood, bringing in men in their role as parents. Mother and child and their health became almost inevitable as a concern to address the persistent high growth of population and low levels of national income (and per capita income) and thus poverty. Healthcare is delivered through a complex system with several providers. Ministry of Health, local self governing authorities, armed forces, social insurance institutions, trade unions, mutual aid societies and co-operatives, charitable and mission institutions, employer-run facilities, private insurance companies, non-government organizations, health management organizations (HMOs), private clinics and hospitals and individual private practitioners including traditional healers. Thus, the main sectors are public or government, social insurance and private.

Locating Mother and Child Health in the Five-Year Plans

The official programme for family planning was launched in 1952 with a budget of 65 lakh rupees, making India the first country to have an official programme and policy for family planning. The concern for MCH was subsumed by the Family Planning Programme (FPP) because of the thrust given to the population growth as a factor responsible for low levels of development. In the Second Five-Year Plan, the allocation for family planning was raised to five crore rupees, while health was given 225 crore rupees. While Bhore Committee (op cit) noted population increase as detrimental to national development and therefore, suggested checks on it through the provisioning of mother and child health-contraception and immunization, the Health Survey and Planning Committee or Mudaliar Committee (GOI, 1961) recommended 'strengthening of the programme to produce early and successful results'. Consequently the Third and the Fourth Plans accorded high priority to family planning programmes and suggested thrust on education and provision of facilities to all populations in rural and urban areas.

Family planning programme as a means to a better economy and health of the women became the core of planned development by the end of the 1950s. The results of the 1961 census showed a higher population growth than expected and gave an impetus to the understanding of the inverse relationship between population growth and development. As a result in the third Plan outlay for family planning was 500 crore rupees and health obtained 342 crore rupees. However, by the end of the Fourth Plan it was realized that family planning approach to poverty had not yielded commensurate results (Cassen, 1978).The strategy adopted for the Fifth Plan was to integrate family planning services with those for health and MCH care and nutrition (GOI, 1974). The vertical programme workers were converted into multi-purpose workers who would pay special attention to family planning for which the outlay was increased to 516 crore rupees while health obtained 797 crores out of the total plan allocation of 53,750 crores. This was 0.95 and 1.49 per cent respectively of the total plan outlay. Poverty was recognized as *'the real enemy'* in the National Population Policy of April 1976. The Policy statement accorded importance to girls' and women's education, nutrition and basic health services. It also reiterated the commitment made in the preceding Fifth Plan to reach a birth rate of 25 per 1000 population by 1984. Rural health services needed to be strengthened to address the poor performance in family planning programme. The Community Health Volunteer scheme was launched in 1977 to tackle the problem of population (GOI, 1980). In the Sixth Five-Year Plan allocation to family planning and health were to the tune of 1010 crores rupees (1.03 per cent) and 1821 crores (1.80 per cent) out of the total outlay of 97555 crores rupees. The Plan acknowledged high morbidity and mortality among children as a cause for 'desire for more children' leading to a high birth rate. Thus for poverty alleviation, nutrition and literacy among women was seen as a means to lower population growth.

The strengthening of rural health services was initiated under the Minimum Basic Needs Programme. It was evident in the Seventh Plan document that performance of MCH component in the field of immunization and ante-natal care was not satisfactory due to factors such as lack of infrastructure, high mortality among infants, children and mother (GOI, 1986). The Plan document recommended strengthening of the health infrastructure and implementation of the family planning programme together with the need to pay greater attention to MCH activities to enhance child survival. The allocation for family planning (3256 crore rupees) was increased to almost equal to health (3392 crore rupees) out of the total budget of 180,000 crore rupees representing 1.8 per cent and 1.88 per cent respectively of the total budget. The Eighth Plan acknowledged that despite being the first country to launch the family planning programme, the birth rates have persistently remained high.

As regards the share of central grants in the state expenditure, there has been a near consistent reduction in medical, public health and family welfare sector from 1984-85 to 1991-92. However, 1992-93 recorded slight increase in all the three sectors. It may be noted that the amount in absolute figures has steadily increased during the same period (Table 1).

Table 1: Central Grants in State Expenditure

Year	Medical	Public Health	Family Welfare
1984-85	6.7	27.9	99.0
1985-86	6.2	26.3	92.1
1986-87	5.0	21.7	90.23
1987-88	4.7	21.4	89.4
1988-89	4.2	19.8	90.9
1989-90	3.9	16.7	74.5
1990-91	3.2	15.2	81.7
1991-92	3.5	15.7	72.3
1992-93	3.7	17.2	88.6

Source: Tulsidhar, V. B., 1994.

Overview of Health Situation

Health of the population appears to be improving as far indicators such as vital rates, life expectancy, and epidemiological indicators such as malaria, leprosy, small-pox, guinea worm and polio. Most morbidity and mortality is caused by preventable and easily curable diseases. Tuberculosis, pneumonia, anaemia, gastroenteritis, dysentery and typhoid together account for 20 per cent of all morbidity. In addition there is large-scale poverty. As far as the epidemiological indicators are concerned, cases of malaria and leprosy have decreased in the last 55 years. Small-pox and guinea worm have been eradicated and polio cases have dramatically reduced from about 30,000 in 1981 to less than 300 in 2000 (Table 2).

Table 2: Changes in Epidemiological Indicators

Epidemiological indicators	1951	1981	2000
Malaria (cases in millions)	75	27	22
Leprosy (cases per 10,000 population)	38.1	57.3	37.4
Small-pox (number of cases)	44887	eradicated	eradicated
Guinea worm (number of cases)	–	39792	eradicated
Polio	–	29709	265

Source: Health Information Statistics of India, 1951; 1981; 2000.GOI.

As regards nutrition, about half of the children aged below five years are moderately or severely malnourished and 47 per cent are underweight. Nearly 30 per cent of newborns are significantly underweight and about 60 per cent of women are underweight.

Protein/energy malnutrition (PEM) is the most common among children below four and iron deficiency/anaemia among those above four and among women (IIPS and Macro International, 2000).

India accounts for one–fifth of the global disease burden with a 17 per cent share of the world's population. India has high levels of deaths due to childhood infectious diseases such as acute lower respiratory infection (28 per cent), diarrhoea (32 per cent), measles (21 per cent) and tetanus (40 per cent). More than 36 per cent population earns less than US$ 1 per day. A fifth of global maternal death and a little less than a quarter of under five mortality (death occurring in children below five years per 1000 live births) occurs in India. Nearly one third of the global burden of tuberculosis and little less than three quarters of the world's leprosy cases are in India. (Table 3).

Table 3: India's Share of World's (ill) Health

India	Percentage of the World
Population	17
People living in poverty (less than US$1)	36
Total deaths	17
Under Five mortality (U5 deaths per 1000 live births)	23
Maternal Deaths	20
DALYs lost	20
Death preventable with childhood vaccination	26
HIV cases	14
Tuberculosis cases	30
Leprosy cases	68

Source: World Bank (2000); WHO (2000).

While India's share of the global burden of disease continues to be higher, some respite comes in the form of decline in death rates of infants, children and adults; and improvements in life expectancy in the last few decades. Life expectancy has nearly doubled during the last 50 years (Table 4).

Regional and social disaggregating of some of the demographic indicators reflects on the variations at these two levels. As regards IMR, national figures pitch at 64 while rural urban differentials range between 40-70 deaths per 100,000 live births. Child (under five) mortality ranges between 63-104 and share of underweight children

Table 4: Demographic Indicators

Indicators	1951	1971	1991	2001
CBR	40	37	30	25
CDR	27	15	9.7	8.1
IMR	146	129	80	63
CMR	25		11	–
MMR	–	500	600	–
TFR	–	5.2	4.0	–
Life Expectancy				
Both	32	46.1	58.2	62
Men	32.5	46.4	58.6	–
Women	31.7	44.7	59.7	–

Note: SRS (Sample Registration System) 2002.

Table 5: Delivery Characteristics and Child Care

Characteristics/Immunisation	1996	2001
Delivery characteristics		
Institutional Delivery	34.0	40.5
Safe Delivery*	40.2	47.6
Child care-Immunisation		
BCG	73	75
DPT3	64	58
OPV3	66	57
Measles	58	56
Full	52	46

***Note:** Either institutional delivery of home delivery assisted by doctor/ANM/nurse
Source: DLHS-RCH 2002-04.

aged <3 ranges between 38-50 per cent respectively for rural and urban populations. Among better performing states in the south, IMR is lowest in Kerala (10) and highest in Maharashtra (45). Similar trends are visible in child mortality, underweight children aged <3 and maternal mortality. Almost all death among children occurs to those aged between 0-4 years. In the rural areas of Orissa, Madhya Pradesh and Uttar Pradesh the infant mortality rate is more than 1000 per 100,000 live births. Higher deaths among girls and women as compared to boys and men up to 35 years and persistently adverse sex ratio are a pointer to the vulnerable health status of women in India. Widespread anaemia and malnutrition combined with poor maternity care services is reflected in high maternal mortality rates ranging from 400 in urban to 800 in some rural parts of the country (IIPS and Macro International, 2002).

As regards social groups, Scheduled Tribes have nearly 56 per cent and Scheduled Castes have 54 per cent underweight children, which is about 8-10 percentage points higher than the national average. Mortality among infants and children is also higher among the tribes as compared to the castes (Table 6).

Table 6: Regional and Social Variation in Health Attainment

India/state	IMR (2002)	U5 mortality (NFHS-2)	%children <3 underweight (2000)	MMR per lakh (2000)
India	64	94.4	47	408
Rural	69	103.7	49.6	–
Urban	40	63.1	38.4	–
Better performing States				
Kerala	10	18.8	27	87
Maharashtra	45	58.1	50	135
Tamil Nadu	44	63.3	37	79
Poor Performing States				
Orissa	87	104.4	54	498
Bihar	61	105.1	54	707
Rajasthan	78	114.9	51	607
UP	80	122.5	52	707
MP	85	137.6	55	498
Social Groups				
India	70	94.9	47	–
Scheduled Castes	83	119.3	53.5	–
Scheduled Tribes	84.2	126.6	55.9	–
Other disadvantaged	76	103.1	47.3	–
Others	61.8	82.6	41.1	–

However, it is noteworthy that though the percentage of poor reduced from 1960s to 2000, the number of poor has increased. Declining trend is visible only after 1979 with an upsurge in the late 1980s and early 1990s largely due to the impact of the economic crisis faced by India then (Table 7).

Poverty is considered to be an important factor contributing towards morbidity and mortality. Communicable diseases,

Table 7: Poverty Trends in India

Year	Number of Poor	% of poor in tot pop
1960-61	17 crores	34
1964-65	22	46
1970-71	25	45
1973-74	32	46
1979-80	**33**	**48**
1986-87	27	34
1987-88	31	39
1993-94	32	36
1996-97	27	29
2000-01	26	26

Source: *Handbook of Statistics* 2002, RBI.

malnutrition and maternal morbidity and mortality are concentrated among poor. Compared to poor (low SLI) rich (high SLI) get sick less and at older ages. The poor experience more than twice as high mortality among infants and children as rich. Also, twice as many poor children are underweight as rich (Table 8).

Table 8: Health Indicators and Standard of Living

Indicators	Low SLI	Medium SLI	High SLI	Ratio low to high
IMR	88.8	70.3	42.7	2.08
CMR	130	94.6	51.5	2.52
TFR	3.4	2.85	2.1	1.60
Children underweight (%)	56.9	46.8	26.8	2.12
Children with anaemia (%)	78.7	73.5	67.3	1.17
Children with ARI (%)	21.0	19.4	15.7	1.34
Children with diarrhoea (%)	19.9	19.7	16.1	1.24
Anaemia among women (%)	60.2	50.3	41.9	1.44

Source: IIPS and Macro International 2000.

Healthcare Service Provisioning

Distribution and training of different types of health personnel and the coverage of health facilities are two important aspects to be considered in understanding care financing. In 1990 there were more than 11000 hospitals, about 28000 dispensaries and 640,000 beds. The rural areas had more than 20,000 PHCs and nearly 131,000 sub-centres (Table 9). While morbidity and mortality trends appear to

Table 9: Gap in Health Services in Urban and Rural Areas

Services	Urban	Rural	Available in Urban	Available in Rural
Hospitals	11,254	2476	Average 3	At the most 1
Dispensaries	27,994	12317	Average 7	At the most 2
Beds	641,615	109075	240 beds*	17 beds*
PHCs	20,641	–	–	2-3
Sub-Centres	130,960	–	–	–

Note: per 100,000 population.

have changed positively over time, healthcare provisioning seems to have failed to keep pace with the requirements. The wide gap that exists in the availability and coverage of healthcare facilities between urban and rural India is glaring. The lopsided thrust on mother and child care has geared almost all finances in the public sector towards it leaving all other services to private care services. It is evident in the organization of health financing and care delivery system.

Priorities assigned to different household members for healthcare utilisation, have age and gender dimensions. The youngest male on the one end of the scale is given the highest priority to the oldest woman with the lowest priority. Within these dynamics is the event and process of child bearing, birth and rearing. Parity and sex of the child is added dimension for locating priorities (Fig. 1). In this regard the two following points may be noted—

1. Public spending on health has been shrinking, forcing the private sector to fill the vacuum, and
2. Since the 1950s, policy recommendations have been to address the 'persistent growth in population' so as to translate the positive impacts of development and usher in 'good health to women'.

Much of the burden of healthcare, therefore, has been with the individual family or household. Given that the burden is higher among the poor, the proportionate expenditure on healthcare too is highest for them.

Sources of Health Finance for Mother and Child

The government (or public) sector provides a broad range of

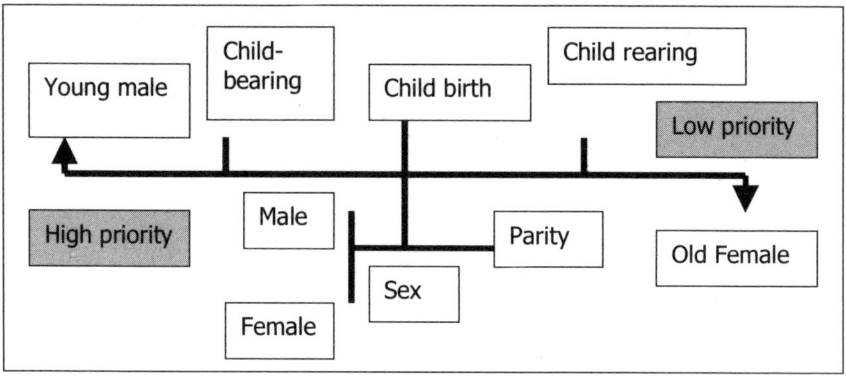

Figure 1: Factors for Prioritizing Healthcare Utilization

services through different programmes run by the Ministry of Health, social welfare, labour, local government authorities and the armed forces. Finance for these programmes is generated from general tax revenue, earmarked taxes, payroll deductions, cost recovery and foreign aid. The state has the responsibility of operating publicly financed healthcare systems through the Ministry of Health with medical care provided at facilities as diverse as referral hospitals at one end and rural health posts at the other. In the 1980s extension of primary healthcare in especially depressed rural areas was emphasised. Decentralisation led to devolution of responsibilities to the local-self government bodies such as municipalities in the urban and panchayats in the rural areas.

General Tax Revenues

Government facilities are supported by general taxation. In low-income countries, duties on imports and exports form the largest component of general tax revenues. Oil exporting countries and those with mineral deposits enjoyed a relative advantage over agriculture-based economies till the 1990s. Taxation of business transactions and profits was another source of income. Such finance was used to support expensive hospital-based programmes that used costly and (often) imported equipments. These hospitals primarily serve the higher income sections, causing inequitable distribution of tax financed health services with facilities concentrated in the urban areas and limited services available to the rural population.

User-fees

A small fraction of revenue is constituted by cost recovery in government facilities. As a welfare state, the government attempted to provide free services to all. Therefore, government health facilities charged no or very little fees for services, drugs and other supplies. However, the economic crisis of 1980s set in motion the health sector reforms which were put in place during the 1990s. Government spending on health declined and cost recovery methods or user fees at government health facilities were instituted during the 1990s. Government health projects covered about 20 per cent of recurrent cost through fees (World Bank, 1987).

Foreign Aid

In developing countries foreign aid accounts for a high proportion of capital costs. Such assistance is often received to expand government healthcare in the rural areas. Funds were also used for recurrent costs of these systems and vertical programmes such as immunization, malaria control and family planning.

Social Security

Most social security systems in health sector provide curative services and cover maternity care. There are two ways through which healthcare is delivered through social insurance—

- In direct method social security institutions have a network of their own hospitals, polyclinics and a salaried health staff through whom medical care is provided to the beneficiaries.
- In indirect method these agencies enter into contract with the physicians and hospitals from the private or public sectors for provisioning of healthcare. Social security institutions may either come under the direct control of the ministries of health or may be autonomous but regulatory by the government.

Private Sector

This sector consists of both commercial and voluntary components and tends to be strong where public services are weak. Commercial health sector constitutes a substantial part of healthcare in India and other developing countries. It covers services sold by both practitioners of modern medicine as well as traditional healers operating from private clinics, offices, hospitals and pharmacies. Government employed physicians may also allot part of their time to private practice. In India, private healthcare sector is 'dominated by individual practitioners, both trained and untrained, at the primary level' (Baru, 2005, 105).

Direct payment in the form of fees is the most common form of payment for healthcare in the private sector. It accounts for more than half of the total expenditure in the developing countries and more than 70 per cent in India during the 1980s. Individual household expenditure on healthcare in the developing countries amounts to two to five per cent of their annual income. In the rural households, the amount is more during the period of poor health. Besides user fees, expenditure on drugs also adds to the spending. The charitable sector also raises finances through user fees. Employer's schemes may directly finance healthcare for their employees by setting up their facilities, by paying for private sector health services through reimbursements, or by entering into contracts with other private institutions/practitioners. Growth of private sector has been governed by the weaknesses of the public sector in delivery of care. Often the reasons put forth for this range from shortage of drugs, inadequate funds, lack of personnel, diagnostic facilities, heavy patient load and unresponsive behaviour of the care providers (*Ibid*. 2005).

Financing of Healthcare

Direct household spending is the largest source of financing healthcare services in India. Reliable data on private health expenditure is not available and, therefore, it is difficult to estimate the volume of household expenditure on healthcare. The official estimate on household consumption expenditure was 56.18 rupees per capita in 1986-87 (NSSO) while the expenditure on healthcare was 45.26 rupees per capita for 1985-86. Some of the household surveys have found that healthcare spending ranges between seven and nine per cent of the household's consumption expenditure. The household expenditure ranges between 175 rupees (Jalgaon, Maharashtra) to 300 rupees (Madhya Pradesh) per capita (Duggal and Amin, 1989; George et al 1993). Such high expenditure in poor countries indicates a very large disease burden and an overwhelming role of the private sector in providing healthcare. In fact, the growth of private sector after 1975 reflects the unmet need for curative care and the failure of the public health system in meeting it. An estimated 88 per cent of household spending on health goes to the private sector. This reflects on the fact that more than three-fourths of the healthcare needs are met by the private sector. Thus, around four per cent of the GDP is contributed directly by households towards their healthcare. A smaller proportion of healthcare finances estimated at 255 rupees are provided by public sources (Nandraj et al. 2001).

The share of health spending in total government expenditure has declined from four per cent in the First Plan (1951-56) to 3.3 per cent by the beginning of the Seventh Plan (1986-90). In addition to this low share of the government, social insurance programmes are also negligible. The share of household expenditure on health has increased both in rural and urban areas during 1994-2000 (Table 10).

There has also been a decline in care use during 1986-87 and 1995-96 in government (public) sources and increase in non-government (private) sources both in the rural and urban areas (Table 11).

Health Expenditure

Health expenditure in India constitutes an estimated six per cent of the GDP. This makes India one of the highest spenders on healthcare in compliance with higher global disease burden. It may be noted that healthcare spending by the government is only 1.4 per cent (much below the WHO recommendation of five per cent) and about five per cent is spent privately by the individual households. This pattern is reverse of the countries where universal and comprehensive healthcare systems are in place. One such country is Norway. Public health expenditure was seven per cent and private was a little over one per cent of the GDP in 2001. Per capita expenditure on health was nearly USD 3000 as compared to USD 80 for India. While Sri Lanka has a balanced share in public(1.8) and private (1.9) health expenditure as percentage of GDP; India's is lopsided with less than one in public sector and more than four in private sector (Table 12). These high levels of expenditure on private healthcare in India are at the cost of essential consumption needs of the poor (Gill and Kavadi, 1999).

Since health is a state subject, 90 per cent of the public spending is accrued through the state budget. Central allocations have slowed down since 1970s and their share in state budget has declined steadily

Table 10: Household Expenditure on Health in Rural and Urban India

R/U	Jul 1994-Jun 1995	Jul 1995 Jun 1996	Jan-Dec 1997	Jul-Dec 1999	Jul 1999 Jun 2000	Jul 2000 Jun 2001	Jul 2001 Jun 2002	Jul-Dec 2002
Rural	4.98	4.07	5.71	5.46	6.09	6.81	6.45	6.76
Urban	3.46	3.73	5.11	5.52	5.06	5.78	5.88	5.77

Source: NSSO 51st to 58th Round.

Table 11: Shift in Care from Public to Private Sector

	Out-patient care				In-patient care			
	Rural		Urban		Rural		Urban	
Source of treatment	1986-87 (42nd Round)	1995-96 (52nd Round)	1986-87 (42nd Round)	1995-96 (52nd Round)	1986-87 (42nd Round)	1995-96 (52nd Round)	1986-87 (42nd Round)	1995-96 (52nd Round)
Pub. Hosp	17.7	11.0	22.6	15.0	55.4	39.9	59.5	41.8
PHC/CHC	4.9	6.0	1.2	1.0	4.3	4.8	0.8	0.9
Pub Disp	2.6	2.0	1.8	2.0	0.0	0.5	0.0	0.4
ESI Doctor	0.4	0.0	1.6	1.0	0.0	0.0	0.0	0.0
All Govt.	25.6	19.0	27.2	19.0	59.7	45.2	60.3	43.1
Pvt. Hosp	15.2	12.0	16.2	16.0	32.0	41.9	29.6	41.0
Nur Home	0.8	3.0	1.2	2.0	4.9	8.0	7.0	11.1
Chart Inst	0.4	0.0	0.8	1.0	1.7	4.0	1.9	4.2
Pvt Doctor	53.0	55.0	51.8	55.0	0.0	0.0	0.0	0.0
Others	5.2	10.0	2.9	7.0	1.7	0.8	1.2	0.6
All Non-Govt.	74.5	80.0	72.9	81.0	4o.3	54.7	39.7	56.9

Source: NSSO 42nd and 52nd Rounds.

(Tulsidhar, 1993) leading to stagnation of public spending and poor quality of rural health services. Healthcare expenditures are categorized as medical, public health, and family welfare. It includes all expenditures incurred by the central and state ministries of health and family welfare (MoH&FW) and expenditure on water supply and sanitation by the ministries of rural and urban development. Private expenditure in health, in fact, has increased both in terms of absolute value in rupees and percentage share of the GDP continuously from 1993-94 to 2002-03 (Table 13).

Table 12: Health Expenditure in some Selected Countries

Country	Health expenditure as % of GDP 2001 Public	Health expenditure as % of GDP 2001 Private	Per capita expenditure on health (PPP US$)
Norway	6.9	1.2	**2920**
USA	6.2	7.7	4887
Malaysia	2.1	1.8	345
Sri Lanka	**1.8**	**1.9**	122
China	2.0	3.4	224
India	**0.9**	**4.2**	**80**
Bangladesh	1.6	2.0	26
Pakistan	1.0	3.0	85

Table 13: Private Expenditure in Health

Pvt Exp	1993-4	1994-5	1995-6	1996-7	1997-8	2000-01	2002-03
billion Rs.	195	279	329	373	459	892	1200
%GDP	2.27	2.75	2.77	2.73	3.00	4.46	4.62

Source: CSO Estimates on Consumption Expenditure 1985 series.

The curative care component in the rural health services is funded through the allocations for public health and family planning. While the private investment in curative care was widely advocated in the Seventh Five-Year Plan (1986-91), public spending was restricted to preventive services. Thus government funds were for selected services such as family planning and child survival programmes at the cost of all other services. While the share of curative services declined in overall expenditures, the family planning (FP) expenditure has grown rapidly since the mid-1960s. The funds in this sector are mostly spent in the rural areas for contraceptives, maternal and child health (MCH) and immunization materials and the salaries of the health workers such as ANMs, MPWs and paramedics based at the sub-centre. For this reason government health services are seen as synonymous with family planning services.

Goals to be Achieved

Some of the goals which have been set to be achieved as millennium development goals include—

- Reduce IMR to 30/1000 and MMR to 100/100000 live births by 2010.
- Increase utilisation of public health facilities from current level of <20 to 75 per cent by 2010.
- Increase health expenditure by government as a percentage of GDP from the existing 0.9 to 2 per cent by 2010.
- Increase share of Central grants to Constitute at least 35 per cent of total health spending by 2010.
- Increase State Sector health spending from 5.5 per cent to 7 per cent of the budget by 2005; further increase to 8 per cent by 2010.

However, given the health sector reforms which have ushered in the regime of privatisation of healthcare, shift from the public to private sector in the care use is evident. Then a larger question which needs to be addressed is that will it be possible to increase public health facility use; health expenditure by government as percentage of GDP and share of central grants to percentage of health spending? The answer could be in affirmative provided careful monitoring of the available care, present system and future needs is done.

Summing Up

As the physical infrastructure of the rural healthcare services was being expanded in the wake of the 1983 National Health Policy, government health spending remained stagnant. MCH and family planning continued to take up maximum share of budgetary allocations and health workers' time. India spends more on health than other developing countries (5-6 per cent of the GDP) but has one of the lowest levels of public financing of healthcare. Increasing public funding appears to be a better alternative to user fees and expansion of private services for a feasible pattern of healthcare financing. It is imperative to ensure quality care to the seekers/users. Paid services need not necessarily be better and therefore may not be actually serving the purpose for which they are introduced.

REFERENCES

1. Baru Rama V., 'Commercialisation of Healthcare—Global and Local Dynamics and Policy Responses' in Mackintosh, M and Koivusalo Meri (eds), Social Policy in Development Context, Palgrave, London, 2005.
2. Berman, P. and M.E. Khan (eds), Paying for India's Healthcare, New Delhi, Sage Publications, 1993.
3. Bhore J., Amesur R.A. and Banerjee A.C., Report of the Health Survey and Development Committee, Vol. I, Government of India Press, New Delhi, 1946.
4. Cassen, R.H., India: Population, Society, Economy, Macmillan, Hong Kong, 1978.
5. Duggal, R. and Amin S., Cost of Healthcare—A Household Survey in an Indian district, Foundation for Research in Community Health, Bombay, 1989.
6. George A. et al. Households Expenditure in Madhya Pradesh, Foundation for Research in Community Health, Mumbai, 1993.
7. Gill Sonya and Kavadi N.S., Health Financing and Costs—A Comparative Study of Trends in Eighteen Countries with Special Reference to India, Foundation for Research in Community Health, Pune/Mumbai, 1999.
8. GOI, Report of the Health Survey and Planning Committee, Government of India Press, New Delhi, 1961.
9. GOI, Planning Commission, Report of the Working Group on Population Policy, Government of India, New Delhi, 1980a.
10. GOI, Planning Commission, Sixth Five-Year Plan, New Delhi, 1980b.
11. GOI, Planning Commission, Seventh Five-Year Plan, New Delhi, 1986.
12. IIPS and ORC Macro International, National Health and Family Survey (NFHS-2), 1998-99, India, International Institute for Population Sciences, Mumbai, 2000.
13. Mitra Asok (1974), 'Population in India's Development' in Bose et al (eds.) Population in India's Development 1947-2000, Vikas Pub, New Delhi.
14. Nandraj S., Madhiwala N., Sinha R., and Jesani Amar, 'Women and Healthcare in Mumbai—A study of morbidity, utilisation and expenditure on healthcare by household of the metropolis', CEHAT—Research Centre of Anusandhan Trust, Mumbai, 2001.
15. Tulsidhar V.B., 'Expenditure Compression and Health Sector Outlays', *Economic and Political Weekly*, 28 (45) Nov 6, 1993.
16. World Bank, Financing Health Services in Developing Countries: A World Bank Policy Study, Washington, IBRD/WB, 1987.

SECTION III

Specific Approaches towards Mother and Child Health

6

Health of Tribal Women and Children: A Holistic and Interdisciplinary Approach

Sunita Reddy

Introduction

Health and health practices are part of the inner most complexities of social existence, permeating the domains of politics, economics and religion and most always connected with dimensions that go beyond the body, such as interpersonal, family and community relationships. Health is at once an end and a means. Medical anthropological studies have built upon historical and cultural analyses over a long period of time that indicates an array of differences with respect to the metaphors and meanings that signify health. These studies have emphasized cultural fabrics that give coherence and depth to these meanings such that cosmology and ethical traditions come to define the body in state of sickness and well being.[1]

Anthropological studies of health focus on local contexts where health and illness are recognized and responded to. Such studies also trace the effects of global flows of commodities, information, finance, images, people and pathogens on such a world. Anthropologists have been as interested in the social roots and consequences of health (and illness) as in their cultural representations. But what most particularly characterizes the anthropological perspective is the use of ethnography to understand health, illness and healthcare. Anthropological perspectives on health brings together individual and collective realities in the way they are organized, narrated, contested and in every sense lived as social trajectories.[2]

What anthropologists learned through research in different societies is a story of diversity in experience of health and healthcare giving as well as the ways social relationships and emotional processes fuse in the medication of health-relevant experiences. The meaning of health ranges from holistic and organic interpretations to hyper-individualistic ones. While biomedicine has treated health as a separate domain, popular meanings and interpretation of healthy states are often inseparable from other moral, political and economic domains. Anthropologists have been particularly concerned with the transformations in health as those transformations express differences in power, social position, and social inequality, particularly as experienced by marginal groups and individuals.[3]

Paul Farmer has shown the ways social forces alter disease distribution and contribute to the persistence of new microbial conditions: indeed, the way social forces and processes come to be embodied as biological events.[4]

Anthropologists have identified the need for cross-cultural studies of health, healing and patterns of morbidity in local contexts. One thread linking these studies is the importance of understanding patterns of everyday life experience, local knowledge and social networks that influence personal agency and access to healthcare, as well as modes of transmission of diseases. From this perspective, health is seen as not simply originating in individuals themselves or deriving strictly from social forces, but as being engendered in complex interactions between individuals and their social contexts. Such lived responses may occur in the context of medical pluralism where several therapeutic systems co-exist in one cultural setting, or in circumstances in which symptoms are subject to several distinct classifications, diagnosis and hence therapeutic courses of action.[5]

Methodology

The present paper is largely based on secondary literature. Apart from the NFHS data, the paper looks into micro level studies on the health of women and children among tribal groups. However, large-scale studies on tribal health status are lacking. Further, desegregated data, on the health of tribal population at national and regional levels too are not available. Due to the scarcity of information, it becomes difficult to get a realistic picture of the health status of the tribal population and more specifically on women and children. This paper is an attempt to bring out the lacunae in information and also address the disparities in the inter-tribe and also intra-tribe health status. The author's field experience among the Konda Reddi tribes of Andhra Pradesh and brief interaction and observations among the primitive tribes of Andaman and Nicobar islands, adds to the content.

Further, the paper tries to look at ethnographic studies, a dominant form of anthropological enquiry, on tribal health and see its strengths and limitations. The 'politics' of ethnographic studies draw attention to the political economy of global inequality that are fore-grounded in ethnographic descriptions.

With the academic background of anthropology and fieldwork done with anthropological perspectives till recently by the author, with a better understanding in public health issues from interdisciplinary and holistic approach now tries to see the same studies and studies done by the other scholars within wider canvas and tries to interlink with wider and larger socio-economic, political context going beyond cultural emphasis. As it is uncertain whether the culture-centric studies can flourish while its practioners remain securely locked up in their academic enclaves. Thus the paper tries to go beyond disciplinary boundaries to analyse the poor health status among the tribal women and children. It also tries to address the heterogeneity among the tribes and their specific health needs.

Composition of Tribes

The tribal population comprising roughly eight per cent of the total population of India numbering around 68 million (excluding Jammu & Kashmir, 1991 census) inhabits widely varying ecological and geo-climatic conditions (hilly, forest, tarai, desert, coastal regions etc.) in different concentrations throughout the country. There are 573 communities recognized by the government as Scheduled Tribes. The extent to which a state's population is tribal varies considerably. In the northeast states of Arunachal Pradesh, Meghalaya, Mizoram and Nagaland, upwards of 90 per cent of the population are tribal. However, in the remaining northeast states of Assam, Manipur, Sikkim and Tripura, tribal people form between 20 and 30 per cent of the population. When compared to these only one per cent of the population of Kerala and Tamil Nadu are tribals, while six per cent of the population in Andhra Pradesh and Karnataka are tribals. The majority of the tribal population, roughly 75 per cent of them reside in central India. The tribes also vary in size with some as big as the Gonds (roughly 7.4 million) and the Santhals (approx. 4.2 million) to as small as the Great Andamanese (45) and the 90-odd Jarawas in Andaman and Nicobar islands.

Most of the Indian tribes are concentrated in varied geographical locations ranging from forests to hills to hill slopes, plains and islands. Most tribes have varied economy from subsistence agriculture, shifting cultivation to hunting and gathering herding, fishing etc. However, due to the rich natural resources in their areas of habitation, they are often displaced for different developmental works, are alienated from their land by the mainlanders and pushed further into poverty, deprivation and dependency.

The tribal people are losing control over their resources due to pressure from more advanced people, displacement by development projects and claims by the state. The tribal sub-plans do provide substantial financial outlays but in the absence of a holistic frame and co-ordinated implementation results have been less than expected.

Thus in order to address the health of women and children from the tribes it is necessary to take into consideration various aspects, their geographical locations, their position in the continuum of development, literacy levels, their economic base, political participation, levels of integration and assimilation and the external agencies and factors impacting their lives.

Health Status of Tribal Women and Children

Maternal and child healthcare is an important aspect of health seeking behaviour, which is largely neglected among the tribal population groups. The planners have to take into consideration the lifestyle, belief, cultural milieu, social organization and channels of communication of the tribal people before introducing developmental activities. The MCH services are almost non-existent and childhood mortality is comparatively high. Comprehensive area-specific health-related studies are limited; most of the available studies are isolated, fragmentary and do not cover the various dimensions of health affecting the status of tribal women. Thus there is a need for proper understanding of their problems specific to time and place so that relevant development programmes can be identified, planned and implemented. It is necessary to take a holistic view from not just a socio-cultural perspective but other economic, ecological and political perspectives.

Early marriage, successive pregnancies accompanied with low calorie of food intake and inaccessibility, unawareness and under-utilization of medical facilities lead to high maternal morbidity and mortality rate. 'Maternal depletion' is thus the result of early mating, continuous cycles of pregnancy and lactation. The inadequate diet and uninterrupted overwork lead to cumulative disorders such as anaemia, general malnutrition, premature aging and early death.

The NFHS II survey provides information on the status of SCs and STs as compared to rest of the population for a number of RCH indicators that are relevant to the Millenium Development Goals. A comparative statement under different RCH components for Scheduled Castes and Scheduled Tribes against the rest of the population is given below.

Health indicator	**SC**	**ST**	**Rest of the Population**
IMR	83.0	84.2	61.8
Child mortality	39.50	46.30	22.20
Under 5 mortality	119.3	126.6	82.6
TFR	3.15	3.06	2.66
% of children underweight	53.5	55.9	41.1
% of children with anaemia	78.3	79.8	72.7
% of children with ARI (prev 2/ 52)	19.6	22.4	18.7
% of children with diarrhoea (prev 2/ 52)	19.8	21.1	19.1
% of women with anaemia	56.0	64.9	47.6

Source: NFHS 1998-99.

Among the standard indicators of health, the IMR is generally considered a crucial indicator of the health status of the population. The IMR, child mortality and under-five mortality were 84.2, 46.30 and 126.6 among the STs in 1998-99 which are quite high as compared to not only the rest of the population but also the SC population. The health status of women also showed that 65 per cent of women suffered from anaemia, and 61 per cent of ST mothers received antenatal check-up as against 80 per cent for others.

Poverty is the prime cause for ill-health, persistent morbidity and early death. However, lack of access to right foods: iron, protein and micro-nutrients such as iodine and vitamins, is the principal cause for the very high incidence of nutritional deficiency diseases: anaemia, diarrhoea, night blindness, goitre, etc. These factors combined with lack of access to basic healthcare services are the main reasons for the unexceptionally adverse differentials in the state of Andhra Pradesh. Under TB and malaria, the tribals suffer disproportionately to their population—the rate of incidence of TB among tribals is estimated to be double and under malaria, case incidence is estimated to be over 18 per 1,000 mostly of the P Falciparum variety, accounting for 75 per cent of the state's total deaths on account of malaria.[6]

Nutritional anaemia is an acute problem for women in India and more so in tribal belt. Tribal women have a heavy workload and anaemia has a profound effect on their psychological and physical health. Anaemia lowers her resistance to fatigue, affects working capacity under conditions of stress and increases susceptibility to other diseases. Maternal malnutrition, which is quite common among tribal women, is also a serious health problem, especially for those having many pregnancies too closely spaced together. It affects the mother's reproductive performance and the birth, which is crucial to the infant's chances of survival and its subsequent growth and development.

Expectant mothers to a large extent were not inoculated against tetanus. Studies have shown that crude birth practices are found in many tribal groups like Kutia Kondhs, Kharias, Gonds, Santhals etc. The main causes of maternal mortality are considered to be unhygienic and primitive practices of parturition, puerperal infection, anaemia, haemorrhage, obstructed labour and sometimes, ruptured uterus.

Most of the tribes are interdependent on their ecosystem of forests, mountains, rivers, and streams and in turn conserve and protect them. The forest-based tribal economy in most parts of the world is women-centred. Food is obtained by shifting cultivation and from minor forest produces (MFP) like flowers and fruits collected from the forest. Extractions from herbs, roots and animals are used for medicines. All these efforts incur excessive workload on women. Because of the extensive felling of trees by vested interests, the distances between the villages and the forest areas have increased forcing the tribal women to walk longer distances in search of minor forest produce and firewood. Given this additional workload even women in advanced stages of pregnancy are required to work in the agricultural fields or walk great distances to collect fuel and minor forest produce. Due to forest protection laws, the tribal populations are given limited area around the settlement for cultivation and cannot go beyond a certain boundary. Cultivating the same area again and again makes it less fertile and with limited technology inputs, reduces the quantity and quality of the produce. As a result of deforestation and the subsequent additional distance to the forest, the availability of food for tribal families has reduced. This has left serious implications particularly for the women who are responsible for the provision and distribution of food. In cases of shortage, they even deprive themselves of food in order to feed others.

Very few women from the tribal areas among Konda Reddis access pre-natal, peri-natal or post-natal care by formal institutions. The birthing is most often home based with a local *dai* or an older woman and sometimes even the husband assisting in delivery. Most often they consult a local *shaman* or folk *healer* and have strong faith in their traditional knowledge. A strong and rich ethno medicine and excellent knowledge of pharmacopoeia have been reported by the Konda Reddis, which is getting lost due to deforestation. Emphasis on family planning has further made tribals become resistant and suspicious about the health services. However, the younger generation women among Konda Reddis intend to have fewer children because of the fear of the painful birthing process while the older women continue to think it is better to have more children as they are not sure of their survival till adulthood. Among the Konda Reddis very few old couples were present and they often practise levirate marriage after the death of the wife, indicating high maternal mortality.[7]

Child Health among Tribes

Three morbidity conditions—fever, acute respiratory infection and diarrhoea—are the most common forms of illness among the ST children. The incidence of anaemia among ST children is quite high, with nearly 78 per cent of them suffering from it. Malnutrition is generally considered as a common disseminator of the disease and deprivation process that reduces child survival. Moreover, malnutrition also results in physical and mental health disorder. Data from NFHS for 1998-99 shows that 26 per cent of ST children fewer than four years of age suffered from malnutrition (based on weight for age). Of these, 56 per cent of ST children were severely undernourished.

Anthropometric measurements to look at various nutritional indices show various grades of nutritional anaemia and Vitamin A deficiency. Unhygienic personal habits and adverse cultural practices relating to child rearing, breastfeeding and weaning practices are seen as the causes for poor health among the tribal children. Tribal children in fact face certain adverse realities like insufficient food intake, frequent infections, and lack of access to health services. Under-nutrition is a well known contributory factor to high mortality in children due to infectious diseases. High infant mortality and under-five mortality rates among Scheduled Tribes have been observed. The problem of under-nutrition amongst pre-school tribal children needs to be addressed through comprehensive preventive, promotional and curative measures. Studies further suggest that the community needs to be educated about environmental sanitation and personal hygienic practices, and also proper child rearing, breastfeeding and weaning practices. However, appropriate nutritional programmes should be designed to meet the requirements. A comprehensive child survival programme with supplementary feeding, growth and development monitoring and early, prompt treatment during illness needs to be devised and implemented ensuring community participation.[8]

Health of Tribes of Andaman and Nicobar Islands

The tribals like Sentinelese, Great Andamanese, Onges are settled in isolated islands, the Sentinel island, Strait island and Little Andaman respectively. As on 2001 out of a total island population of 356,265, there are only 92 Onge, 43 Great Andamanese, 350 Jarawa,, 100 Sentinelese and over 250 Shompens who constitute primitive tribes (Sircar, 2004). The livelihoods of most of the tribals are based on forests, which have been encroached, and some developmental programmes like the construction of Andaman Truck Road (ATR).

The Jarawas heartland has been torn apart for building the ATR. The 340 km long ATR from Port Blair in South Andaman to Diglipur in North has been constructed through the heart of the very forests the Jarawa call home and the Tribal Reserve. This road has increased access to the Jarawas and poses the greatest threat to them as well as the forest that they have protected for so many years. After the Jarawas have come out of their isolation, this road has greatly increased contact with outsiders resulting in the most damaging impact on their lives. 57 miles of the ATR passes through the Jarawa Reserve area (Sekhsaria, 2003).[9]

Further, the policies to integrate the tribals, like the 'contact programme' with Jarawas, Onges, and Great Andmanaese have proved to be disastrous from an anthropologist point of view. These contact programmes are criticized the most for intruding into their lives, natural habitats, bringing new addictions like alcohol, gutka and tobacco and introducing various diseases and sexual exploitation. Addiction to alcoholism by the tribals is now used by settlers to exploit forest produce. Poaching and encroachment inside the Onge reserve, too, are ever on the increase. Tribal people have incredible knowledge of the forests and the sea. Insensitive development policies and logging operations have brought them to the brink of extinction today.

Micro-level studies among the tribes of Andaman and Nicobar islands show the rich resources the tribes have in terms of forests and the forest produce. The nutrition of Nicobarese, currently numbering around 30,000,[10] consists of coconut, pandanus, wild pig, megapode, marine fauna, etc. which are abundantly available throughout the Nicobarese. MML (Manulo Matai Limited) canteen, Pilobhabi, supplies ration to all households throughout the year. There is no scarcity of food but marine fauna are less available during rainy season. Coconut is one of the main items as well as source of income among the Nicobarese. Pandanus, coconut and raw milled rice are consumed daily by all households. Pork or fish is also consumed at least thrice in a week. Nutritional anthropometric data indicates the physique of a Nicobarese male as quite satisfactory. However, according to weight/height index, 25 per cent of women are categorized as undernourished. According to the pignet index 8.07 per cent of women are categorized under 'very weak' physique. Though obesity is common in both the sexes, few among the

Nicobarese are anaemic. The overall haemoglobin concentration in the blood is unsatisfactory, though severe anaemia could not be found among them. However, intake of calories, protein, iron and vitamins are low in comparison to ICMR recommended value but intake of fat and calcium exceeds ICMR recommended allowances.[11]

A demographic and health profile of the Jarawas was carried out.[12] The derived ratios/indices of the height and weight of the studied samples indicate that among the adult males 60 per cent were in the normal state of nutrition and 12 per cent were moderately overweight. However, only 28 per cent adult males showed a tendency towards a very mild under-nutrition to low state of malnutrition. Among women, about 70 per cent were in the normal state of nutrition and 20 per cent were moderately overweight individuals. Only six per cent of the adult women indicated a very mild under-nutritional state of health. Among the children (23 individuals, 15 boys and 8 girls, 4-12 years of age) about 20 per cent boys and 25percent girls indicated a low state of under- nutrition.

The Jarawa tribe has been surviving in the jungles of Andaman for thousands of years with their traditional medicine system. Medical coverage through mobile dispensary twice a week at different camps treated respiratory tract infections, skin diseases, ulcers on their bodies and worm infestations. Jarawas have been coming to Kadamtala PHC since September 1997. After coming into contact with the settled people, the Jarawas used to suffer from different types of infections. In June 1999, assessment of Jarawa health problems showed that 42 of them were suffering from respiratory tract infections. Jarawas know good anti-diarrhoea medicines and their food hygiene is very good. They are known to prevent mosquito bites during night by applying an herbal juice over their bodies. Jarawas never come for ante and post-natal care and for confinement of any new born child. During post-natal period, mothers are found to be healthy and without any anaemia problems. It was reported that they had no hypertension, congenital disease, dental caries, or thyroid disorders and cases of malnutrition were almost nil.[13] In October 1999 and more recently in May 2006, Jarawas suffered from measles infection and that could have happened due to their mingling with their neighbours. On 21st Sep. 1999, 23 Jarawa patients from PHC Kadamtala were brought to the G.B. Pant hospital. Fifty-two cases from Kadamtala and 90 cases in Port Blair—half of the estimated Jarawa population suffered from measles, pneumonia, acute upper and lower respiratory tract infections and fungal infection of skin.[14]

Once predominant, the Great Andamanese tribe was decimated due to epidemic diseases introduced inadvertently by outsiders who established their penal settlement colony during the nineteenth century. The population of the Great Andamanese was around 5000 prior to the arrival of the British in the Andaman to find the penal settlement of Port Blair. They founded an Andamanese home here and according to old government reports, a syphilis epidemic wreaked havoc among the Andamanese and nearly destroyed them. Syphilis was followed by ophthalmia and then in 1877, measles and pneumonia and influenza together with the widely spread syphilis rendered a devastating blow to the demographic stability of the Great Andamanese. In 1985-87, epidemic dysentery took its toll among the Shompens. The toll could not be checked among the Shompens because of their accessibility and lack of planning to meet such a medical exigency. Malaria is no less devastating. Malaria might have been prevalent only among the Nicobarese who inhabit the coastal region. However, with the beginning of economic intercourse between the Shompens and Nicobarese, the former may have contracted malaria. Health is a crucial aspect for the survival of a small community like the Shompens. Shompens have their own ethno-medicine to meet the requirements which had been in use for generations. However, it is the epidemic diseases caused due to contact with outsiders which have turned out to be a nightmare to the Shompens as it would to any other small isolated communities.[15]

The above literature shows that the nutritional levels of the tribes in the Andaman and Nicobar islands is far better due to the forest resources, access to sea and also government doles provided to them. However, of serious concern are their dwindling numbers and the threat of extinction due to the diseases contracted by their contact with outsiders. The health problems of the tribes in the Andaman and Nicobar islands are different from the other tribes in the mainland where poverty and food scarcity are the major concern.

Interdisciplinary Approach

Maternal mortality is reported to be high among various tribal groups but desegregated data is not available. Studies on maternal and child healthcare practices are largely neglected in various tribal groups. Most of the anthropological ethnographic studies done are micro-level and gives very enriching insights into the etiology, perceptions of people regarding their illnesses, cultural practices and magico-religious practices related to the various rites of passage ceremonies, starting from birth to menstruation, marriage, child birth to death. Most of these studies on women and children's health gives vivid descriptions of childbirth practices, child rearing practices, the customs and ceremonies attached to all these occasions and weaning practices. Most often these studies come up with factors behind their ill-health as unhygienic practices, lack of awareness, fatalistic or irrational unscientific views, illiteracy, and not seeking proper medical care. Thus they are usually reductionist and blame the victims and culture. Very few studies have gone beyond these culture-centric approaches and behavioural recommendations and linked ill-health to larger economic, political, ecological and developmental issues. Rarely have the studies been linked to the non-availability, unaffordability and inaccessibility of healthcare and hardly any study has linked these to the doctor-patient relationships. Especially when the whole hospital set-up, service providers and purely biomedical approach make the tribals feel alienated and threatened.

The issues of power differential and 'competence gap' between doctors and patients, medical dominance, the vulnerability of patients and their capacity for resistance is hardly studied with respect to the tribal population. A problem with the functionalist analyses of power in the medical encounter has been their tendency to focus on the micro properties of the interaction between doctors and patients without analyzing the social and political context in which such encounters take place. The political economy approach views medical dominance as the outcome of a power struggle among a number of different interest groups, each of them intent on achieving high status and power. Political economists argue that there is a social class schism between doctors and patients which acts to preserve power on the side of doctors in the medical encounter. It is possible that people of a lower social class may feel at worst alienated and at best intimidated by the doctor's air of authority and omnipotence.[16] The tribals with the lowest social class in the hierarchy with all the disadvantages of poverty, illiteracy, and lack of political power are bound to feel alienated in the modern medical set-up. The tribal women are doubly disadvantaged as there are no lady doctors in the dispensaries. Other paramedical staff like the ANMs or other multipurpose workers too possessing power and status are inaccessible to the tribal people.

The non-utilization, alienation and non-compliance by the tribal population have to be understood not as an individual problem, ignorance or the resistance by the tribal population towards modern medicine. It needs to be seen from the larger context of social status of the tribals in the social hierarchy and the power differentials between the doctor or health worker and the tribal patient. Further studies need to be done on these aspects of healthcare delivery and acceptance of the people.

It has been recognized that there are barriers to accessing services because of various factors. The causes are many like poor connectivity to health centres because of distance, topography, and lack of public transport, location disadvantage of sub-centres, PHCs, CHCs, social and cultural barriers especially for women, and lack of suitable transport facility for quick referral of emergency cases. From the service provider's side lack of accommodation, poor infrastructure, large-scale absenteeism and vacancies, poorly trained and unmotivated manpower are the reasons for the near-absence of healthcare services. Due to poor working environment and lack of incentives to work in remote areas, service providers do not feel motivated to work. This further adds to the weak monitoring and supervision system.

Tribal health in the Tenth Plan document ensures adequate access to healthcare services for the tribal population, with 20,769 SCs, 3286 PHCs, 541 CHCs, 142 hospitals, 78 mobile clinics and 2305 dispensaries already established in tribal areas. Under the National Anti-Malaria Programme (NAMP) 100 identified predominantly tribal districts in Andhra Pradesh, Bihar, Gujarat, Madhya Pradesh, Maharashtra, Orissa and Rajasthan are covered. In spite of all these, the access to, and utilization of, healthcare remain suboptimal and health and nutrition indices in the tribal population continue to be poor.[17]

Among the experiments for improving access to primary healthcare among tribals, in Orissa, additional central assistance is provided for mobile health units with a fixed tour schedule. In

Karnataka and Maharashtra, NGOs have adopted and are running PHCs in tribal areas. The success of all these experiments is mainly due to the commitment of individuals and credibility of NGOs, which are difficult to replicate.

Challenges

There is no desegregated data on the health status of the tribal population, health outcome measures, and data on health indicators. However, a few small-scale or micro-studies now and then give a profile of the tribes and their health conditions. In other cases it is brought to the limelight when there is breaking news or sensationalized reports about starvation deaths among children, in several interior pockets though it may be a recurring phenomenon all the time.

Very few studies have tried to link poor health status and deprivation to the issues of poverty, unemployment, lack of access to income earning capital assets, heavy dependence on wage employment, high unemployment, low education, less diversification of employment and other factors. None has suggested the need to make necessary modifications in the policies to improve the ownership of income earning capital assets, employment, human resources and health situation.[18]

The health of tribal women has to be looked at from a need-based approach as women in various tribes pursue various economic activities. Women in the forest areas are more prone to accidents, fatigue, undernourishment and maternal depletion. Women who are in the nomadic and de-notified tribes, being mobile, need different strategies to cater to their health. Tribal women who are migrating to cities, like those from Jharkhand and other tribal belts, may be victims of abuse by their employers or need special attention. Women who are pushed into sex trade like those from the Kanjar tribe on the roadside have entirely different health needs. In the continuum of development, some tribes like the Khasis of the northeast and the Meena of Rajasthan are economically better off with higher literacy levels when compared to most other tribes, where the educational levels are low and they are economically deprived.

With the developmental activities and opening up of the tribal areas for tourism, it is necessary to understand its impact on the lives of the tribal people. The tribals are lured to exchange forest produce for alcohol which has led to alcoholism among the tribes of Andaman and Nicobar, especially the Great Andamanese and Jarawas. Further, the tribal women are sexually exploited. The situation has come to such a pass that the Jarawa tribe people have started begging on the roads which pass through their scheduled area. Further opening of these tribal areas to tourism in many places across states whether in Jharkand, Chattisgarh, Nilgiri Hills or Andaman and Nicobar islands is going to bring in various vices and ill-health among the tribal women. It is reported that the RTI and STI have been contracted from outside in these islands. It is to be explored how far the developmental activities have brought economic gains and what losses they have incurred.

Because of the heterogeneity in the tribal population their health needs too will differ. Conflict, be it ethnic conflict in the northeast, or naxal conflict in Orissa, Madhya Pradesh and parts of Andhra Pradesh have serious implications for the mental health of the people who live there especially the poor and disadvantaged like the tribals. Women who are forced into drug and sex trafficking have separate health needs from women who are migrating to urban areas. How to address the health needs of such a population is a major challenge with maximum limitations in place.

The limited studies among the tribals and their health are due to various reasons, starting from lack of funds to logistical problems and very few anthropologists who are willing to study the remote and inaccessible areas.

Looking Ahead

In retrospect it becomes clear that the studies focusing on behaviour and culture are not going to go too far in improving the health of women and children in the tribal areas. In order to improve the health status of the tribals, it is necessary to have a holistic view of their living conditions and bring women to the centre-stage of development. Safe drinking water, roads, electricity, schools and functional, affordable health services have to be provided in the vicinity. It is also necessary to ensure livelihoods and food security to the tribals especially women and children. We further need to ensure and protect their rights over the forest and other natural resources in their areas.

It is imperative to take cognizance of the tribal situation vis-à-vis their ecosystem. There is an immediate need to recognize and protect the traditional knowledge, customs, and practices of indigenous people. Further, ethno-botanical investigation and scientific enquiry to preserve their knowledge should be carried out and there should be a stop to their valuable source of knowledge from vanishing. In order to reduce the burden of women in collecting firewood, focus should be on increasing the biomass in nature and conservation of biodiversity. Women should be fully involved in decision- making and in the implementation of sustainable development activities. Priority should be given to gender-sensitive, participatory, action-oriented research and policy analysis. Measures should be taken to develop and include environmental, social and gender impact analysis as an essential step in the development and monitoring of programmes and policies. Thus, it can be summed up that there is a need for a holistic approach to environment, economy, energy, equity and development.[19]

There are many urgent issues, which need attention. Detailed information is needed on maternal malnutrition, nutritional anaemia, nutritional status of pregnant women and their nature of workload, the distribution of food within the family and its effect on the nutritional status of women, the complications of pregnancy and childbirth, practices for parturition, maternal mortality, birth weight of children, infant and childhood mortality and their sex differentials, nature of maternal and child healthcare practices, attitude towards family planning etc.

There is a need to document the levels of poverty, levels of deprivation, nutritional status, food security, unemployment, housing, wages, access to land, forest, water resources, access to safe drinking water and electricity within the tribes as the tribes too are heterogeneous.

Tribal development strategies will need to be more human-centred. This means having an agenda that consists of provisioning of basic education, basic healthcare, and capacity building within the framework of a stable and sustainable land use policy, where there is a basic inter-linkage of the individual activities. It also means better targeting so as to ensure an equitable development processs. The development paradigm will need to make health centre-stage in the overall development strategy.[20]

The primary healthcare for tribal areas must be conceived and planned anew. The priority problems must be decided based on the disease pattern of the concerned tribal population. Problems like accidents, burns, sickle cell disease, malaria, T.B., leprosy, sexually transmitted disease, endemic, goitre may need special attention.

Trained workers from outside shall not become stable in the tribal areas, so the workers must be selected from among the tribals and trained. Indigenous systems of healthcare and indigenous practioners should be incorporated in healthcare planning. Greater role for voluntary organization is required. Further anthropological and comprehensive approaches are essential for enhancing our understanding of the health problems of women and children and help them to plan their own healthcare.

In order to generate a data bank, compilation of all the micro studies both published and unpublished in various states should be compiled. A national survey should be conducted to produce desegregated data on the health conditions of various tribes. More research studies should be carried out to see the implications of rampant tourism in the scheduled areas on the health of women and children.

Stringent and strict laws should be made and implemented to protect the rights of the tribal people. Policies related to use of forest lands and health of the tribes should be favourable to the tribes.

NOTES

1. International Encyclopaedia of the Social and Behavioral Sciences, Vol. 10, Smelser Neil J., and Baltes Paul B., Elsevier, Oxford, 2001.
2. Kleinman A., Writing at the Margin: Discourse Between Anthropology and Medicine, University of California Press, Berkely CA, 1995.
3. International Encyclopaedia of the Social and Behavioral Sciences, Vol. 10, Smelser Neil J., and Baltes Paul B., Elsevier, Oxford, 2001.
4. Farmer P., Infections and Inequalities: The Modern Plagues, University of California Press, Berkeley, CA, P.5, 1999.
5. Leslie and Young, Paths to Asian Medical Knowledge, University of California Press, Berkeley, CA, 1992.
6. Rao Sujata K., 'Healthcare Services in Tribal Areas of Andhra Pradesh: A Public Policy Perspective', *Economic and Political Weekly*, 33 (9). Feb. 28-March 6, 1998. pp. 481-486.
7. Reddy Sunita, 'Childbirth and Child Rearing Practices among Konda Reddi Tribes of Andhra Pradesh', *Man in India*, 2002.
8. Rao V.G., Yadav Rajeev, Dolla C.K., Kumar Surendra et.al, 'Under Nutrition and Childhood Morbidities among Tribal Preschool Children', *Indian J. Med. Res.* 122, July 2005, pp. 43-47

9. Sheksaria P., Troubled Islands, Kalpavriksh Lead—India, 2003.
10. According to census of 2001, the Nicobar Islands have a total population of 42,026, including settlers and Shompens.
11. Chattopadhyay M. and Ravi Prasad B.V., 'The nutritional status of Nicobarese of Great Nicobar Islands', in Tyagi D. and Bhattachary K.K., *Nutritional Status of Indian Population: Andaman and Nicobar Islands,* Anthropological Survey of India, Ministry of Tourism and Culture, Department of Culture, GOI, Kolkata, 2003.
12. Sarkar B.N., and Sahani R., 'A Demographic and Health Profile of the Jarawas of the Andaman Islanders', pp. 132-147 in Mukhopadhyay R. K. (ed) *Jarawa Contact: Ours with Them Theirs With Us.* (Bhattacharya, Sarkar B.N, Anthropological Survey of India, Ministry of Tourism and Culture, Department of Culture, GOI, 2002.
13. Kar R.C., 'Medical Coverage Provided to the Jarawas—A note on the basis of personal experience' pp. 148-154, in Mukhopadhyay K., Bhattacharya R.K., Sarkar B.N., (eds) *Jarawa Contact: Ours with Them Theirs with Us,* Anthropological Survey of India, Ministry of Tourism and Culture, Department of Culture, GOI, 2002.
14. Mathews E., 'Health Problems and Healthcare of the Jarawas in the Transition Phase', pp. 155-160, in Mukhopadhyay K., Bhattacharya R.K., Sarkar B.N., (eds) *Jarawa Contact: Ours with Them Theirs with Us,* Anthropological Survey of India, Ministry of Tourism and Culture, Department of Culture, GOI, 2002.
15. Awaradi S.A., Master Plan (1991-2021) for Welfare of Primitive Tribes of Andaman and Nicobar Islands, A & N Administration, Port Blair, 1990.
16. Lupton Deborah, Medicne as Culture, pp. 113-119, Sage Publication, Delhi, 2003.
17. Government of India (2002a): Tenth Five Year Plan. New Delhi, *Planning Commission*. pp. 81-164.
18 . Thorat S.K., Empowering Marginalized Groups—Policies and Change, p. 72, India Social Development Council for Social Development, OUP.
19. Reddy Sunita, 'Ecosystems Approach to Human Health: A Case of Konda Reddi Tribes of Women's Health', *J. Hum.Ecol,* 16 (4):271-282 (2004).
20. Rao Sujata K., 'Healthcare Services in Tribal Areas of Andhra Pradesh: A Public Policy Perspective', *Economic and Political Weekly,* pp. 481-486, 33 (9), Feb. 28-March 6, 1998.

7

Mothers and Children Affected by HIV/AIDS in India: Issues and Concerns

Dr. R.R. Gangakhedkar

Background

HIV infection being a sexually transmitted disease classically spreads in three waves. Sex workers constitute the first wave. When HIV infection establishes itself among clients of sex workers and the spouses and children of clients of sex workers, the epidemic is presumed to have reached the second and third wave respectively. Typically, women are at the centre of the epidemic initially and also in the third wave. The issues among women differ by their level of empowerment. Certain issues are more likely to be different among mothers who are sex workers over those who belong to mainstream population. The major challenges for providing preventive, curative and other services to women and children are poor health and treatment seeking behaviour, lack of availability of affordable prevention tools such as condoms or vaginal microbicides, low income generational skills among women, inadequate/exploitative responses faced by widowed woman, non-availability of paediatric formulations of antiretroviral drugs, continuing resistance to take an infected baby for foster care and host of other social issues.

Magnitude

The first few cases of HIV infection were detected among sex workers from Chennai in 1986 in India. According to the National AIDS Control Organisation, it is estimated that 5.1 million individuals were infected by HIV in India at the end of 2004. Of the, two million women estimated to be infected by HIV, about 1.2 million live in rural areas. The male-to-female ratio among those who are infected by HIV is estimated to be 1.56:1 whereas among reported AIDS cases it is 2.42:1 at the end of July 2005. According to the National AIDS Control Organisation (Sentinel Surveillance Data, NACO 2004), the HIV reactivity rates among pregnant women in five Indian states—Maharashtra, Karnataka, Andhra Pradesh, Manipur and Nagaland—have reached more than one per cent, a sign of a well-established epidemic in the low risk population. HIV estimates released by NACO in 2004 have not segregated paediatric HIV infections. With 27 million pregnancies and an overall estimated 0.88 per cent prevalence rate of HIV infection among pregnant women and a transmission rate of 30 per cent, about 70,000 infants will acquire HIV infection from their mothers every year in India.

Natural History of HIV Infection Among Women

The rate of HIV disease progression is known to depend on the viral set point in the first year of HIV infection. The higher the plasma viral load, the lower is the incubation period. Later, the HIV disease progression can be predicted by the rate of decline of CD4 lymphocytes each year. A few studies have shown that women tend to have lower plasma viral loads than men for a similar CD4 count when compared to men. This finding implies that antiretroviral therapy should be initiated at a higher value of CD4 counts than the generally accepted cut-off between 200 to 250 cells per cumm. However, a similar finding was not reported in other studies. The guidelines to treat with ART continue to be similar for men and women, globally. Women tend to have a higher CD4 count when they seek consultation for the first time for symptomatic HIV disease as compared to men. A study done in south India reveals that the median CD4 count among such women is 358 cells per cumm compared to 162 cells per cu mm among men. However, this can best be attributed to the fact that women are likely to be evaluated early as their husbands' HIV disease status tends to influence the treatment-seeking behaviours. Therefore, the median survival was found to be about three times higher than that among men. Women are more likely to seek care for recurrent candidal vaginitis and pelvic inflammatory disease. Human Papilloma Virus infection manifesting as genital warts is an important condition for management among women. HIV infected women are two times more likely to develop cervical cancers once they develop cervical abnormalities. Though the virologic response to antiretroviral therapy is not different between genders, certain side-effects are likely to be more frequent or severe among women. Lactic acidosis, lipodystrophy and gastro-intestinal symptoms such as nausea, vomiting and diarrhoea are more common among women compared to men.

Prevention of Mother-to-Child Transmission (PMTCT)

The efficiency of mother-to-child transmission (MTCT) of HIV-1 ranged from seven per cent to 13 per cent in Europe, about 25 per cent in the United States, and up to 40 per cent in Africa. A study reported that the efficiency of MTCT was reported to be 48 per cent in India. A wide variety of factors have been attributed for the variations in MTCT in different geographic areas. The efficiency of MTCT of HIV-2 was reported to be 1.2 per cent when compared to 24.7 per cent of HIV-1 that is almost 20 times lesser than that of HIV-1. HIV transmission can occur during intrauterine, intrapartum, and post-partum period. The important determinants that enhance the risk of MTCT of HIV-1 are clinically advanced disease or primary HIV infection, type of delivery—vaginal and c-section for obstetric indications, premature rupture of membrane, presence of co-factors like chorioaminionitis, sexually transmitted diseases (STDs), cracked nipple, breast abscess, and breast-feeding.

There are four major approaches to reduce PTCT. The first approach aims at reduction of the maternal viral load by using antiretroviral drugs. The second focuses towards reducing the exposure of the foetus during intrapartum period to HIV through offer of elective c-section and avoidance of invasive obstetric practices such as use of forceps, episiotomy and foetal blood samples from scalp for estimating pH. The third attempts to foster safer infant feeding practices and the last approach works over promotion of primary and secondary prevention strategies against HIV infection. The first study to reduce mother-to-child transmission of HIV infection using three part zidovudine regimen (PACTG 076) reduced the transmission rate by about 67 per cent from 25.5 per cent to 8.3

per cent in a non-breast-fed setting. In 1998, a CDC-Thai study that aimed at shortening the duration of administration of zidovudine by providing zidovudine 300 mg twice a day from 36 weeks gestation onwards and 300 mg three hourly during labour was found to reduce the risk of transmission by 51 per cent from 18.9 per cent to 9.4 per cent. In 1999, single dose nevirapine to pregnant woman during labour and to the newborn within 72 hours of birth (HIVNET 012) when compared to a short zidovudine regimen reduced the risk of transmission by 47 per cent from 25.1 per cent to 13.1 per cent at 14-16 weeks after birth. Since HIVNET 012 regime was simple to offer, could potentially enhance coverage and provided almost equal reduction in transmission rates, a decision to use it in scaling up PPTCT strategies in India was made in 2001.

Between January-December 2004, about 11, 34,000 pregnant women were registered in 288 PPTCT centres of which about 83 per cent (9, 40,000) received counselling. Of those who were counselled, about 88 per cent accepted HIV test. About 8000 pregnant women were found to be infected by HIV. During the same period, about 2, 11,000 women (17 per cent) came directly in labour. Of those who came in labour and could be tested, 1872 women were found to be HIV infected. Of the total (registered plus those directly coming in labour) 4451 mother-newborn pairs could be offered SD NVP. Of the registered women who were counselled, 77 per cent came back to collect their HIV test results.

Though single dose nevirapine approach is simple, cheap, less toxic and fairly effective approach, a few publications have reported development of nevirapine resistant mutations among 22 per cent to 70 per cent women as well as their HIV-infected babies. The first report tended to suggest that it develops among 22 per cent women who received SD NVP at 6-8 weeks post-natally and the drug resistant mutants disappear by 12 months. However, the disappearance of drug resistant mutations may also be due to archiving of the resistant virus and inability of the current assays to detect them. A recent study used highly sensitive methods and found that up to 70 per cent women and about 50 per cent of their babies who had acquired infection show presence of drug resistant HIV. These mutations are associated with development of class resistance that affects not only use of nevirapine but also efavirenz when the mother needs ART for management of her advanced HIV disease. It is also known that emergence of drug-resistance is likely to be more common in HIV-1 sub-type C which is the predominant subtype in India. The first evidence suggesting that provision of SD NVP limits maternal therapeutic options came from a landmark study published from Thailand in 2004.

It reported that development of nevirapine resistant mutations was associated with lower proportions of women achieving virologic suppression at six months when they needed ART and were provided NVP-based ART. The current free ART programme in India relies on provision of nevirapine or efavirenz-based ART. Nevirapine/efavirenz-based three drug combination is cheaper, less toxic and almost as effective as any other combination regimen in managing advanced HIV disease. If a woman develops NVP resistant HIV infection, she can potentially transmit it to her husband through unsafe sex. Such persons will require first-line antiretroviral therapy using non-NNRTI containing regimen, the cheapest of which may cost about six times higher than nevirapine-containing regimen. Additionally, these regimens are more toxic than NVP based regimens.

Issues and Concerns: Management of HIV Disease

(a) Early diagnosis of HIV infection

Though voluntary counselling and testing for HIV infection was one of the first activities undertaken, the coverage and its acceptance were low especially so for women. Provision of single dose nevirapine to reduce PPTCT was accorded a high priority in six high HIV prevalence states in India. There was a fear that it may lead to a 'blaming others' syndrome in the family and may have an adverse social impact on the infected women. Strategies to promote partner testing were promoted in PPTCT programme. Though there is no evidence to suggest that women faced marital discord, the partner testing rates continued to remain low. The increasing coverage of PPTCT will bring in infected women early for medical consultations and thus enhance quality of life and survival among women. But the frequency of domestic violence is high in India. In absence of large published studies, it is difficult to say whether it would increase and can be attributed to woman being the index case.

(b) Management of HIV disease using ART

Prior to initiation of free ART programme, HIV physicians used to report that those on ART are mostly males, a reflection of male dominance in the society and differences in HIV disease staging among males and females. This difference was minimized when a priority was accorded to women with advanced HIV disease who had received PPTCT interventions. However, the emergence of nevirapine resistant HIV after receipt of single dose nevirapine in a large proportion of women is a major concern. Not only does it limit therapeutic options for women but may also lead to the development of a drug resistant HIV epidemic. Realising the importance of emergence of NNRTI resistance, the National AIDS Control Organisation is planning to use different regimens to reduce parent-to-child transmission. However, even when a simple nevirapine based regimen was being used, the coverage of antenatal women for PPTCT was only about four per cent. There is a major concern that use of complex regimens may complicate the issues further. However, it is also necessary to weigh the benefits and challenges associated with each of these approaches which warrant a change in regimen.

(c) Treatment seeking behaviour and drug adherence

Traditionally treatment seeking behaviour among women is impacted by her immediate environment. With free ART programmes in place, the proportions of women accessing care has increased especially since her husband is more likely to be attending these clinics, the concerns were minimized considerably. However, the situation becomes complicated among widows. The mother who has uninfected child/children is more likely to be having good treatment seeking behaviour. However, if the child is infected, the health of her baby is more likely to be accorded a high priority and neglect of personal health is observed commonly (personal experiences). Death of an infected child is also associated with extended grief and a long period of indifference to her own health issues that become a major challenge in a woman receiving ART. Strategies that involve a family member as medicine providers or supervisors need to be implemented. After the death of her husband a large proportion of mothers are brought back to her parent's house as 'retaliation' or a 'protective' response. Mothers of a younger age group housed with old parents having limited income can also pose a major challenge in seeking care.

(d) Social discrimination

Most often women tend to face discrimination at family level than men. Women are likely to be blamed for infecting their husbands, sent back to their parents and are likely to be not able to exercise their rights over the property. Provision of legal assistance is a critical need among widows. Younger uninfected women are likely to be exposed to sexual exploitation. If marriage is a risk factor for acquiring HIV infection, re-marrying remains a safer option for many of them. Though there are some reports of marriages among two infected persons in certain parts of Maharashtra, it is still in initial stages of a response.

(e) Child bearing

There is an immense social pressure on HIV negative women in HIV discordant couple settings. The low empowerment of women and perceived social expectations about motherhood affects her ability to balance risks appropriately. The couple is likely to 'mutually' agree to resort to having unprotected sex. Those who are infected continue to worry about whether she will be 'lucky' and have a baby that is not infected. Sometimes this concern may make her almost paranoid. The access to antiretrovirals can often be limited due to the social tradition of her movement to her parent's place for delivery.

Natural History of HIV in Children

Most of the HIV natural history cohorts in children have shown that there is a bimodal distribution of clinical disease progression. These are classified as rapid progressors and slow progressors. Of the HIV infected children, about 20-30 per cent are rapid progressors. The rapid progressors tend to develop advanced disease usually in the first year of life (mostly by five to six months of age). About 50 per cent of these children develop AIDS by five years of age. Majority of infants not treated with antiretroviral drugs maintain a very high burden of viral load.

Majority of the paediatric HIV infection cases can be categorised as slow progressors. These children are relatively asymptomatic during infancy and according to a study about 15 per cent were asymptomatic even at five years of age. The slow progressors generally tend to have higher CD8 counts and reveal a lower rate of fall of absolute CD4 counts. About one-fourth of these children may show mild symptoms such as lymphadenitis and parotitis.

There are certain differences between HIV- infected children and adults such as:

1. Children infected with HIV tend to have a lower survival span
2. Their virological and immunological responses tend to be different from adults
3. They tend to have a different morbidity profile than adults
4. They are more likely to have growth retardation and generalised systemic manifestations such as hepatosplenomegaly etc.

The pharmacokinetic profile of drugs is different in children. The bioavailability of any drug is especially a critical issue in management. One needs to pay attention to the nutritional aspects especially the food-drug interaction. The non-availability of paediatric formulation of various antiretroviral preparations poses a major hurdle in management. Immunisation of infants appropriately is critical in paediatric HIV management. All these issues make paediatric HIV management a complicated task.

Issues and Concerns

(a) Early diagnosis

Many studies have shown that early diagnosis of HIV infection among children is critical in enhancing survival as it picks up those who are early progressors. HIV ELISA detects presence of antibodies against HIV. It has a limited utility in early diagnosis as maternal antibodies against HIV are passively transferred to the baby during pregnancy. These antibodies disappear around 15 months of age. Therefore, use of two HIV-1 DNA PCR—first between one to two months of age and the second six weeks after stopping breast feeding or if the baby is not breast fed, after four months of age is necessary. However, the test is sophisticated and costly. The National AIDS

Control Organisation is planning to devise strategies to enhance access to PCR technology.

(b) Management of HIV disease in children

The rapid progressors among children are likely to develop potentially fatal pneumocystis jiroveci pneumonitis. In order to prevent it, cotrimoxazole prophylaxis needs to be initiated at six to eight weeks age of babies born to HIV infected mothers and continued until sero-reversion is detected. However, the coverage of cotrimoxazole is low in India. Reorienting paediatricians to enhance coverage is vital in reducing infant mortality due to this pneumonia.

US FDA has approved 21 antiretroviral drugs so far for human use. Unfortunately, the pharmaceutical companies test these drugs among adults and are not keen to test them in children as the number of infected children is smaller globally. Therefore, very few antiretrovirals with paediatric formulations are available. These drugs are mentioned in the following table:

Availability of Paediatric Formulations!

(Colour red if only out-side India; India is supplier of the world if colour Green)

- Nucleoside Reverse Transcriptase Inhibitors *(NRTIs)*
  - *<u>Zidovudine (ZDV)</u>* ***Didanosine (ddI)*** *Zalcitabane (ddC)*
  - *<u>Lamivudine (3TC)</u>* *<u>Stavudine (d4T)</u>* ***Abacavir (ABC)***
  - *Emtricitabane (FTC)*
- Non-nucleoside Reverse Transcriptase Inhibitors *(NNRTIs)*
  - Nevirapine (NVP) *Delavirdine (DLV)* *<u>Efavirenz (EFV)</u>*
- Nucleotide Reverse Transcriptase Inhibitor
  - *Tenofavir*
- Fusin Inhibitor - ***Enfuvirtide***
- Protease Inhibitors *(PIs)*
  - *Indinavir (IDV)* ***Ritonavir (RTV)*** *Saquinavir (SQV)*
  - ***Nelfinavir (NFV)*** ***Amprenavir (AMP)*** *Atazanavir*
  - ***Lopinavir (Kaletra)***

The low availability of paediatric formulations limits therapeutic options in infected children. Worse still, if the baby fails on the first line, provision of second line antiretrovirals becomes extremely difficult as the formulations that are available are adult formulations (larger doses). Though use of antiretrovirals is not associated with severe side-effects as in adults, use of higher doses as a helpless response is not an ideal situation. It is necessary to advocate with pharmaceuticals and also legislate as in US that any new drug that is registered for use among adults must start trials in children as well. Unless this issue is addressed, enhancing survival is going to be an extremely difficult task as the dosages in children need repeated adjustments as their weight increases. Most often physicians treat children as mini adults and reduce dosages arbitrarily. This needs to be avoided.

Adherence to medicines is an important issue. Most often parents need to be informed well about the importance of drug adherence. Coincidental symptoms can often lead to drug defaulting as it is likely to be attributed to the medicines.

(c) Orphan child

A large proportion of these children become orphans. Most often they land up with their grandparents. However, their age and limited income have an adverse impact on children, especially on their nutritional needs.

Foster care needs to be preferred over admission in orphanages. However, foster care option for infected children is yet to be accepted well when compared to the uninfected babies. HIV test is offered to all the babies in orphanages before adoption. Adoption during infancy is always promoted. However, most of those who are HIV ELISA reactive may eventually sero-revert. But, prospective parents most often find it difficult to accept such children as normal children.

(d) Disclosure issues

Some HIV infected children reach adolescence. Some of them also require antiretrovirals for management as they grow older. The children may insist that they need to know why they need to take medicines every day. The disclosures of HIV status is a sensitive issue and needs to be tailored by their level of comprehension and maturity. Most often, the fear is that accidental disclosure of sero-status may occur through the child resulting in discrimination. However, hiding the status may pose major difficulties later on.

(e) Discrimination in schools is also common

Their admission to schools could be denied and an infected child could even be expelled from school. Training the school management is a critical step to avoid discrimination in schools. This is also vital as school absenteeism is common in infected children due to repeated illnesses. Some of them could be slow learners. These issues need to be handled sensitively by the schools.

Programmatic Response

HIV infection has evoked social stigma as a community response in all walks of life that was also seen in the past to tuberculosis, leprosy or syphilis. The stigma tends to be higher for sexually transmitted infections and more so for males. Even the development and implementation of prevention and control programmes face a major challenge in such infections. However, overall socio-economic development brings in the social recognition of women and children as the most vulnerable sub-populations. Interestingly, programmes that focus on women and children become an entry point to strengthen the strategies especially those addressing the empowered males in the society. National STD Control Programme is one of oldest national programmes in India that had expanded only up to clinical service provision up to district level through sexually transmitted disease clinics in pre-HIV era. The first of the targeted interventions began among female sex workers around 1989 and later they were followed by other sub-population such as truckers, men having sex with men and other bridge populations such as migrants etc... Even in treatment strategies primacy was accorded to provide counselling that in addition to other issues emphasized the issues surrounding partner management in persons having sexually transmitted diseases and strengthen efforts to reduce missed opportunities to treat among women attending gynaecology out-patient departments through trainings. Prevention of mother-to-child transmission programme was the first programme that was based on use of antiretrovirals (2001). Even the free antiretroviral therapy programme in India had the first inclusion criteria as women and children who had received antiretrovirals for prevention of mother-to-child transmission! To address the issue of stigma, the name was also changed to Prevention of Parent-to-child Programme. Thus women and children affected by HIV have posed major challenges but have also provided us opportunities to initiate comprehensive quality interventions to all the subpopulations including males against HIV.

Conclusions

Mothers and children affected by HIV pose a major challenge for the health system. The prevention of mother-to-child transmission strategies based on simple feasible single dose nevirapine is likely to limit maternal and paediatric therapeutic options. Paediatric HIV infection poses challenges while treating with antiretrovirals due to the non-availability of paediatric formulations. Both mothers and children are likely to experience serious social discrimination. On the positive side, strategies to reduce impact among mothers and children have greatly helped in initiating comprehensive programmes.

REFERENCES

1. Farzadegan H., Hoover D.R., Astemborski J, Lyles C.M., Margolick J.B., Markham R.B., et al, 'Sex differences in HIV-1 viral load and progression to AIDS', *Lancet*, 352:1510-4, 1998.
2. Rezza G., Lepri A.C., d'Arminio Monforte A., Pezzoti P., Castelli F, Dianzani F., et al, 'Plasma viral load concentrations in women and men from different exposure categories and with known duration of infection', I.CO.N.A Study Group, *J. Acquir Immune Defic Syndr*. 2000, 25:56-62.
3. Anastos K., Gange S.J., Lau B., Weiser B., Detels R., Giorgi J.V. et al, 'Association of race and gender with HIV-1 RNA levels and immunologic progression', *J. Acquir Immune Defic Syndr*, 2000, 24:218-26.
4. Bush C.E., Donovan R.M., Markowitz N., Baxa D., Kvale P., Suravolatz L.D., 'Gender is not a factor in serum human immunodeficiency virus type 1 RNA levels in patients with viraemia', *J Clin Microbiol*, 1996;34:970-72.
5. Moore R.D., Cheever I., Keruly J.C., Chaisson R.E., 'Lack of sex difference in CD4 to HIV-1 RNA viral load ration' (Letter), *Lancet* 1999; 353:463-64.
6. Kumarasamy N., Solomon Suniti, Flanigan Timothy P., Hemlatha R., Thyagarajan S.P., and Meyer Kenneth, Natural History of Human Immunodeficiency Virus Disease in India, *Clin Infect Dis* 2003; 36:79-85.

SECTION IV

Institutional Framework of Health Service: Issues of Power, Responsibility and Accountability

8

A Red Herring: Population Policies and Maternal Health in Neo-Liberal Times

Prof. Mohan Rao

Close to the dawn of Independence, the Indian National Congress established the National Planning Committee in 1938, under the chairmanship of Jawaharlal Nehru to outline the shape of India's tryst with destiny and to contour it. One of the sub-committees, chaired by Col. Sokhey, was devoted to the question of health policy. The Sub-Committee on Health also considered, quite naturally, the question of population and maternal and child health. At a time when no nation in the world sponsored a family planning programme, Laksmibai Rajwade forcefully argued the case for the inclusion of "birth control, provision of goods, instructions, demonstrations and consultations" in maternal and child health services. Birth control, she argued:

> "... is obviously a very important function in view of the fact that the high mortality among mothers and children is in part due to too frequent pregnancies involving a terrific strain on the nerves and on a vitality already abnormally low. Children are born not as a creative evolutionary response to the vital urge, but as brittle standardised products of a tired reproductive machinery automatically set in motion by the sexual act. The reproductive system has to be kept fresh and vitalised to respond creatively and must not therefore be subjected to that strain. That can only be done by controlling pregnancy by contraceptive methods." (NPC 1948:133)[1]

Calling for the creation of a "comprehensive medical service financed wholly by the State available to all persons" (NPC 1948: 158)[2], Rajwade pointed out that "to keep up the interplay of life and death about 20 mothers have to starve or poison themselves to death for every thousand of births; that out of the thousand born at such awful cost nearly 175 to 200 die before they are a year old; that on the scarred survivors of this stupendous ordeal is laid the responsibility of reproducing and building up their race in this land" (NPC 1948: 119).[3]

The National Planning Committee's Sub Committee on Women's Role in Planned Economy resolved:

> "The health programme of the state shall aim at the eradication of serious diseases, more especially such as are communicable or transmissible by marriage. The state should follow a eugenic programme to make the race physically and mentally healthy. This would discourage marriages of unfit persons and provide for the sterilization of persons suffering from transmissible diseases of a serious nature, such as insanity or epilepsy (NPC 1948:114)."[8]

Thus are tied together familiar if disparate themes: the health of the 'race' and the nation, the health of women and children, and the health of the population. What is also immediately apparent is that the yoking together of women's health with that of reproduction has a long history. What is also extremely interesting is that in this discourse the troubled, indeed fraught ideas of Indian womanhood that had informed a range of nationalist debates in the nineteenth century, from age of consent to sati, had been eclipsed. In the colonial period Indian women had been objects of nationalist reformist agendas setting right what were conceived as the aberrations of the recent past; practices such as widow immolation and child marriages were evidence to the British that they did indeed have a civilizing mission among the barbaric and traditional Hindus. Extremely contentious debates had arisen about the new or modern Indian woman to be brought into being in a new Indian nation; a woman who was to be distinguished both from the materialistic un-godly Western woman and the common Indian woman, superstitious and sexually promiscuous (Chatterjee and Riley 2001).[4] This modern woman was to be a good woman, a chaste wife, a good mother, enlightened yet spiritual, who would participate in nation-building through harnessing children as resources. The nation state itself was conceived of as a body composed of physically and morally healthy citizens to which all must contribute (Zachariah 2001).[5] This could only be achieved through reproductive prudence, harnessing bodies for a sublime and sublimating nation-state.

In the unanimity that prevailed about the need for population control, two remarkable men however stand out sharply, Mahatma Gandhi and Periyar. Gandhi was opposed to birth control because he believed that society would be enervated, weakened, by birth control. "The sex urge", he wrote, "is a fine and noble thing...but it is meant only for the act of creation. Any other use of it is a sin against God and humanity" (cited in Srinivasan 1995:18).[6] He dismissed Margaret Sanger's arguments for contraception on the grounds that it increased self-indulgence. Thus he wrote:

> "It is certain that excessive indulgence increases the rate of infant mortality. People in the West limit births, not with any religious idea, to be sure, but for reasons of health and for fear of having to bring up too many children. For us such is not enough...We in India lay great claim to being more religious in our lives than people in the West, and yet we ignore the restraints imposed by religion. Hence it is that many parents, regardless of both dharma and worldly considerations, remain steeped in carnal pleasures and bring forth children regardless of circumstances. The result, whether we want them or not, diseased children are born and die in their infancy" (Gandhi: 1920:469).[7]

When Sanger wrote to him, pleading for birth control on the grounds of the suffering imposed on women by frequent pregnancies, he was rigidly unbending, befitting a patriarch of a Hindu joint family. He replied:

> "I agree that there are hard cases. Else, birth control enthusiasts would have no case. But I would say, 'Go and devise remedies by all means, but the remedies should be other than the ones you advise'. I carry on correspondence with many of these people and they describe their ailments to me. I simply say that if I were to present them with this method of birth control, they would lead far worse lives" (cited in Srinivasan 1995: 19).[8]

That he did influence the national Sub-committee on Woman's Role in Planned Economy is evident in their compromised observation:

> "Self-control is the best method for those who can exercise it without ill-effects to their health. But this is a method which we cannot offer to the average man and woman and hence knowledge of scientific methods of birth control must be made available for those who desire it"(NPC 1948:203).[9]

Periyar's views, far ahead of his times, and thus perhaps ignored, were strikingly at variance. He rejected eugenic and neo-Malthusian arguments on entirely rational grounds, but equally strongly argued for birth control for women, to enable them to control their own lives, to break servitude to patriarchy, to caste and indeed the family. Thus he wrote:

> "There is a fundamental difference between our reasons for the necessity of contraception and those of others. That is, we say, contraception is essential for women to be free and autonomous. They say it is essential for women's health, national economy and to prevent fragmentation and destruction of family property. First of all, whether a woman needs birth control or not should be entirely woman's decision. Secondly, the objective of birth control is not to control the growing population or to advance the economy, but to create an environment for women to have rights and decision-making power" (cited in Anandhi 2000: 155).[10]

In the event, of course, neither Periyar, who adumbrates with startling relevance indeed with contemporaenity, nor Gandhi's views, influenced policy. We find thus two compelling—if not necessarily complementary—concerns shaping the emerging population policy. The first relates to the benefits accruing to national development, what is to become the familiar neo-Malthusian refrain; and the second, to the benefits accruing to women's health through birth control. While not contesting the latter, it is nevertheless important to note that this emphasis on women as reproductive beings whose "tired reproductive machinery is automatically set in motion by reproductive act", is an abiding concern with policy-makers. This concern does three things: first, it focuses on women primarily as reproducers, ignoring all their myriad productive activities that indeed contribute to national development. Second, it serves to isolate reproduction from the socio-economic context within which it occurs. Finally, it also serves to draw attention away from the huge non-reproductive causes of mortality and morbidity among women.

Over the years, then, concern for women's health has been expressed through two programmes, the MCH programme and the family planning programme. Thus women are conceived of as merely reproductive beings, whose reproduction threatens their own health and the health of the nation. Over the years too family planning programme has set the agenda for health in general, contouring and inhibiting health sector development (Rao, 2004).[11] As a result even MCH services have been severely neglected. The National Population Policy 2000 (NPP) is said to have moved away from narrowly focused demographic concerns to issues of women's health and reproductive rights. This paper seeks to examine how far we have gone in this "paradigm shift".

I

On the 30th of July 2003, a three-judge Bench of the Supreme Court of India upheld a Haryana Government law prohibiting a person from contesting or holding the post of a sarpanch or panch in the PRIs of the state if he or she had more than two children. The Bench observed that "disqualification on the right to contest an election for having more than two living children does not contravene any fundamental right, nor does it cross the limits of reasonability. Rather, it is a disqualification conceptually devised in the national interest" (Venkatesan 2003:1).[12]

Interestingly, while the Supreme Court spoke about the "torrential increase of population", earlier the Rajasthan High Court judges, hearing a similar set of petitions, in their ruling argued: "These provisions have been enacted by the legislature to *control the menace of population explosion*... The government is spending large sums of money propagating family planning. One of the agencies to which the project of family planning has been entrusted for implementation is the gram panchayat. The panches and sarpanches are to set the example and maintain the norm of two children. Otherwise what examples can they set before the public?" (Sarkar and Ramanathan 2002:42).[13] More recently, on 28th February 2005, in response to a Public Interest Litigation (PIL) petition filed by an NGO in Rajasthan pleading for the implementation of the two-child norm at all levels, the Supreme Court issued notices to the Centre and the states on the implementation of the two-child norm (Press Trust of India 2005).[14]

Haryana is not the only state that has a population policy with such features, which are not only at variance with the NPP but also strike at the heart of the commitments to reproductive health and rights made by the government at the ICPD. Other states, such as Andhra Pradesh, Madhya Pradesh, Rajasthan, Chattisgarh, Himachal Pradesh and Uttar Pradesh, also carry this policy prescription in their population policies.[20] Between them they also advocate a mind-boggling host of incentives and disincentives: restricting schooling in government schools to two children; restricting employment in public services to those with two children; linking financial assistance to PRIs for development activities and anti-poverty programmes with performance in family planning; linking assessment of public health staff to performance in family planning and so forth. Indeed service rules for government employees have been altered in several states making a two-child norm mandatory.

Many of these state population policies—such as those of Andhra Pradesh, Rajasthan and Uttar Pradesh—were drafted, it must be noted, with the assistance of a consultancy firm from the United States named Futures Group. This firm has a distinguished record of creating fears of "population explosion" among policy-makers in Africa in order to initiate population control programmes (Hartmann 1995).[15] Most of these policy prescriptions were mooted, often on the advice of foreign experts, in the population bomb and Cold War years of the early sixties and found expression in the Minority Report of the Mudaliar Committee in 1961. They found expression on the field for the first time in the days of the Emergency.

The Supreme Court ruling has come in for widespread middle-class approbation. Indeed, the Supreme Court ruling perhaps renders redundant some of the private members' bills in Parliament that have been tabled to variously increase incentives or disincentives. Two of them, one named the Population Stabilisation Bill, 1999 (Lok Sabha Secretariat 1999),[16] and the other, the Population Control Bill 2000 (Lok Sabha Secretariat 2000),[17] for instance, moot the idea of a one-child norm along with a number of incentives and disincentives, including disqualification of persons with more than one child from contesting elections. Yet another bill, the Bachelor's Allowance Bill 2000, suggests incentives to those men who remain bachelors (Lok Sabha Secretariat 2000).[18] Men, who, after taking advantage of the incentives, subsequently get married, are to be fined and imprisoned. Yet another bill, the Population Control Bill, 2000, also seeks to punish people who violate the small family norm with rigorous imprisonment for a term of five years and a fine, not less than 50,000 rupees (Lok Sabha Secretariat 2000).[19] The Population Control and Family Welfare Bill, 1999, proposes in addition to incentives and disincentives, the compulsory sterilization of every married couple having two or more living children (Lok Sabha Secretariat 1999).[20] The State Law Commission of Uttar Pradesh drafted the Uttar Pradesh Population Control Bill, 2002 (Government of Uttar Pradesh 2002)[21] This Bill codifies all the anti-human rights features of the State Population Policies, with a slew of disincentives for "any person who shall be deemed to have committed a breach of the family planning norm if he has more than two living children, one of whom is born on or after the appointed date" (Government of UP. 2002:1). These include disqualification from employment and promotion, disqualification from membership in any co-operative union, housing society, public corporation and so on, denial of bonus, honorarium or any other benefit, denial of increments, denial of housing loans etc. Failure to inform the authorities of the birth of a child in violation of the norm would invite disciplinary action, including dismissal from employment.

It would perhaps not be out of place to note the uncanny similarities between some of the measures proposed in the state population policies and the World Bank's pronouncements in its influential document, *India's Family Welfare Programme: Towards a Reproductive and Child Health Approach* (Measham and Heaver 1995).[22] Although the Bank was one of the major actors shaping the Cairo consensus (Rao 2004),[23] when it came to India's programme, it remains unconverted. Having paid obeisance to the concept of reproductive health, and the transformation to India's family planning programme this would harbinger, the Bank argues:

> "The new consensus recognizes that an important goal of reproductive health programmes should be to reduce unwanted fertility safely, thereby responding to the needs of individuals for high quality services, as well as to *demographic objectives*" (The World Bank 1995: 14).

Thus is a mountain of hope and optimism transformed into a lowly molehill. The very heart of the idea of reproductive health mooted by feminists – that there should be no over-riding demographic goals – is torn out in this avatar of reproductive health. In this transformation, "the agenda of reproductive health is seem as a method of attaining demographic objectives set by faceless financial institutions and governments" (Sengupta 1998: 34).[24]

This conceptual revisionism achieved, the Bank—which actually used the discredited phrases 'population explosion' and 'control of population'—set out all too familiar strategies. What is remarkable about this document is the weaving in of the same old concerns, albeit in the light of ICPD.

> "FWP could ... offer panchayats financial incentives to take reproductive and child health initiatives (Ibid: 39).
>
> Targets based on micro-level planning suiting the local specific needs may, however, continue to be fixed for monitoring of the programme (Ibid: 50).
>
> An innovative package of incentives/disincentives be formulated with emphasis on community based incentives and social security measures for individuals adopting the small family norm The community based incentives would be linked to various benefits being made available to the public under different socio-economic development plans of the government (Ibid: 50).
>
> No more incentive to government employees will be considered. A suitable package of disincentives will be developed for this section of the society for adoption by the state governments as well. It will also be recommended to the employers in the organized sector (Ibid: 50).
>
> In order to give a wider choice of contraceptives to the acceptors, new contraceptives such as Norplant-6 and injectables shall be introduced under the programme, initially under controlled conditions and gradually on a wider scale" (Ibid: 51).

Further embellishments are of course for a greater role for the private and NGO sectors, and, in an increasingly communal atmosphere, "religious leaders at different levels" (Ibid: 48). The bottomline, as they say, is that "de-linking of programmes from demographic objectives does not imply that slowing of population growth should cease to be a goal of the population policy" (Ibid: 58).

It is not, then, surprising that efforts at prescribing a two-child norm seem to be found in amazingly unlikely quarters. The Tamil Nadu Agricultural Labourer's Insurance Bill, for instance, stipulates that labourers losing their limbs can only receive insurance compensation if they have no more than two children. Recently, the Maharashtra government passed a law for differential irrigation fees; farmers with more than two children would be required to pay more for irrigation facilities (*The Hindu* 2005).[25] More creatively, the U.P. government announced a scheme whereby applicants for gun licenses had to produce certificates that they had motivated five cases for sterilization (Sharma 2004).[26] More recently still, a delegation from the Indian Medical Association has urged the government to, following China and implement a One Child Norm (Kurup 2005).[27] In yet another move, also recalling the days of the Emergency, in Rajasthan, school teachers have been given sterilization targets to achieve.

In short, then, there is widespread political consensus, cutting across party lines, that the population question is alarming, and that there should be greater "political will" in tackling this issue on a priority basis. This is shared by and large by the elites and middle classes in general, from the media to the judiciary and the medical profession. This is singularly ironic for two reasons. First, as signalled by the NPP, it was precisely during this period that efforts were made to bring about a "paradigm shift" in population discourse in the country, to move away from demographically driven population concerns. Second, it was particularly during these years that the government had in fact shed, or whittled down, whatever commitments it had for social issues and the welfare of the poor as it embraced unbridled free-market policies at the behest of international funding agencies, and in meeting the demands of India's vocal middle class, now increasingly "seceding" from the nation.

Not to be left behind, the Government of India announced in April 2003 its plans to introduce in the Lok Sabha the Constitutional (79th Amendment) Bill seeking to restrict persons with more than two children from contesting elections (*The Hindustan Times* 2003).[28] This Bill, introduced in the Rajya Sabha in 1992, would first have to pass the lower house. The Health Minister, speaking in the Lok Sabha, announced that should there be consensus on the Bill, the government was prepared to introduce it in the ongoing session of Parliament, before elections intervened and the Government was swept out of power.

What is also immediately apparent in all these policy initiatives that the original *raison d'être* for population policy—the health of women—has utterly receded from the foreground. Instead, the NPP notwithstanding, the focus is on controlling women's reproduction. At the same time with the macro-economic policies of liberalization being followed since the 1990s, state commitment to health has declined.

As a result, what we find today is improvements in infant and child survival of the range anticipated, and indeed that the 1990s, with the onset of liberalization, have seen their stagnation. The rate of decline of the IMR and U5MR has sharply decelerated. The percentage decline in IMR between 1971-81 was 14.7; between 1981-91 it was even more marked at 27.3 per cent. However in the period 1991-99, there has been a marked stagnation with the rate of decline in the IMR at 10 per cent. While there has been a decline in the U5MR, the pace of decline has come down and is currently hovering around 95 per cent. During 1971-81, the percentage decline was 20.6. The decline was much sharper during the eighties, with a percentage decline of 35.7. However during the nineties, with the onset of policies of liberalisation, the rate of decline has reduced to 15.1 per cent (Misra *et al* 2003).[29] Along with the shrinking of funds for public health and the concentration on vertical programmes, to the neglect of general health services, one singular feature is what can be described as the family planning approach to health sector development. Thus it has been goals in family planning that have contoured health sector development in the country.

This is evident from the financial allocations made over the years to health and family planning. While allocations to health have shown a secular decline, those towards family planning have shown a proportionate increase. Thus commencing in the First Plan with a minuscule 0.1 per cent of the budget, when health obtained 3.3 per cent, the allocations to family planning increased to 1.5 per cent in the Eighth, when health obtained 1.75 per cent and to 1.8 per cent in the Ninth when health obtained 1.1 per cent. At the same time expenditure on MCH has declined over the years (Qadeer 1998).[30] As the NHP notes, health spending in India has declined to 0.9 per cent, substantially less than spent on health, on average, even in the countries of sub-Saharan Africa (1.7 per cent). Indeed the only countries with less public spending on health are Myanmar, Sierra Leone, Georgia, Kampuchea and Congo. The pursuit of targets in family planning and the priority that has been accorded to it has meant that other aspects of healthcare have been neglected, including the provision of MCH services. Thus it is not surprising that the NFHS-2 results show that "mothers in India received ante-natal check-ups for only 65 per cent of births during the three years preceding the survey, almost unchanged from 64 per cent in NFHS-1". (NFHS 200:282).[31] Indeed considering all the components of ANC, the NFHS-2 notes that "for India as a whole, mothers of only 20 per cent of births received all the components of antenatal care" (*ibid*: 305). It is not surprising too that communicable diseases and anaemia continue to be predominant causes of maternal deaths.

As many as 130,000 mothers die during childbirth every year. The NHP 1983 target for 2000 was to reduce Maternal Mortality Rate to less than 200 per 100,000 live births by 2000. However, 407 mothers die due to pregnancy-related causes, for every 100,000 live births even today. As per the NFHS, between the two rounds in the nineties, the MMR has increased from 424 to 540 maternal deaths per 100,000 live births. High, and unconscionable as these levels of maternal mortality are, it is nevertheless critical to bear in mind that they represent just a fraction of the morbidity and mortality load borne by women in the country. Thus, for instance, deaths due to anaemia among women who are not pregnant are twice as much as among those who are. Similarly, communicable diseases take a much higher toll than those due to pregnancy and childbirth.

So overwhelming has been the influence of targets in the programme that pursuit of sterilization goals to the neglect of health occurs even today despite an apparent official commitment to a target-free approach. Thus women and children, and indeed men, are denied essential healthcare even as the PHC system is geared towards meeting family planning targets (Menon 2004).[32] Indeed even abortion services are not accessed by women seeking them primarily because they are tied to family planning, sterilization in particular (van Hollen 2004).[33] The preoccupation with family planning targets also means that women from the Muslim community, seeking healthcare including contraception, do not access the PHC system for fear of sterilization (Jeffery and Jeffery 2006).[34]

Thus the entire PHC system has been suborned for family planning, distorting its priorities and programmes. Both the NPP and the Ninth Plan document recognize that there is large need to augment and strengthen healthcare services and to meet the unmet needs for contraception. Indeed the Ninth Plan document also noted that one of the priorities for the programme would be to reduce high wanted fertility due to prevailing high IMR that is estimated to contribute 20 per cent to the population growth rate, while the unmet need for contraception contributes another 20 per cent (GOI undated).[35]

Clearly then, given this realization, policy initiatives relying on incentives and disincentives are unnecessary, if not absurd. But what is also ignored is the larger context that frames both health and population policy.

As we noted earlier, while state commitment to the public sector has declined—we have had what can only be described as state-led collapse of the public health system—the state has provided impetus to the growth of the private sector in healthcare through a range of subsidies and schemes (Baru 1998).[36] Thus India has the largest and least regulated private healthcare system in the world.

The collapse of the public health system, without which of course the RCH approach cannot be implemented, has meant that increasing numbers of the poor are thrown at the door of the private medical care sector. The NCAER study reveals a per capita annual out-of-pocket health expenditure of 170 rupees. While there is gender parity at lower levels of expenditure, higher levels of expenditure are associated with marked gender disparities. Higher levels of gender differentials in health expenditure are also evident in the 0-4 year age group. Although the richer classes spend more in absolute terms, they spend an insignificant amount in relation to their household incomes. The poorest spend substantially more proportionate to their incomes. It is thus not surprising that even as healthcare becomes more inaccessible, expenditure on healthcare is emerging as the leading cause of indebtedness (Krishnan 1999).[37] At the same time, reports of starvation deaths and outbreaks of epidemics have started pouring in (Baru and Sadhna 2000).[38]

The NCAER study therefore concludes: "Cuts in public expenditure as a result of structural adjustment and privatisation of healthcare will adversely affect the poor and vulnerable" (Sharif 1999:148).[39] The conclusion then is inescapable: that reforms which bypass vast sections of the population cannot but be accompanied by stagnation, if not deceleration of health indices, among these sections.

Inter-regional, rural-urban, gender and economic class differentials in access to healthcare in India have been fairly well documented. But since the onset of liberalization policies, these have considerably widened. State support for private healthcare grew with the initiation of private-public partnerships that took a variety of forms. At the same time, there were far-reaching changes in drug policies. Thus India—earlier characterised by relatively low costs of drugs and pharmaceuticals, along with a significant indigenous production of drugs—has witnessed a greater concentration of drug production, a larger role for multinationals, a higher proportion of imported drugs and unbelievably steep rises in the costs of drugs (Sengupta 1996).[40] Concurrently, marked shifts have occurred in healthcare utilisation. Among people who sought out-patient services in 1995-96, more than 80 per cent did so in the private sector, a sharp increase in even the poorer states of the country (Sen, *et al* 2002).[41] In 1995-96, 55 per cent and 57 per cent in rural and urban areas were hospitalized in the private sector compared to 40 per cent in 1986-87. NSS data indicates greater inequality in use of health facilities by economic class gradients. In rural areas the class gradient in in-patient use of public hospitals–which was insignificant in the mid-1980s—turned statistically significant in the mid-nineties. In urban areas, inequality in use of public facilities did not worsen significantly, but inequality in use of private facilities did. The steep fall in rural hospitalization rates, along with increasing use by the better-off indicates that the poor are being squeezed out. Fee-for-services is undoubtedly one important mechanism that has succeeded in doing this. In other words, World Bank policies on health, contained in the *World Development Report, 1993,* succeeded in doing exactly the opposite of what was ostensibly its *raison d'etre*: reduce the utilization of public services by the better-off to increase access to the poor.

Costs of both out-patient and in-patient care increased sharply in both rural and urban areas, compared to the mid-eighties. Private out-patient costs increased by 142 per cent as against 77 per cent in the public sector in rural areas. In urban areas, private out-patient costs increased by 150 per cent compared to 124 per cent in the public sector. The increase in costs in in-patient care is even more striking:

average costs rose by 436 per cent in rural and 320 per cent in urban areas (Sen *et al* 2002).[42] Thus it is that even the NHP (2002) notes that medical expenditure has emerged as one of the leading causes of indebtedness (GOI 2002).[43] At the same time, the proportion of people not availing *any type* of medical care due to financial reasons increased between 1986-87 and 1995-96: from 10 to 21 per cent in urban areas, and from 15 to 24 per cent in rural areas (GOI 2000).[44]

It is often argued that one reason why the government has introduced expenditure cuts is that there is a squeeze on government finances. What is not highlighted is that over the nineties the government is either less willing or unwilling to collect taxes even at levels that existed before the onset of reforms. Thus the tax GDP ratio has declined from more than 13 per cent in 1980-81 to 9 per cent in 2000-2001. At the same time, of course, this implies that regressive indirect taxes as a proportion of revenue has increased, taxes paid for disproportionately by the poor. But just the reduction in direct taxes represents uncollected revenues of 4 per cent of GDP, which is almost three times the entire expenditure on public health, medicine and family welfare by the central and state governments combined.

One reason for the growing neglect of women's health issues, along with the anti-poor thrust of neo-liberal policies, I would suggest, is also the profound anti-feminisms of the period. Along with the spread of Hindutva ideologies, and indeed other fundamentalist ideologies, all of which have sharply increased around the world in this period of neo-liberal reforms, state policies are also actively contributing to the reinforcement of anti-female ideologies and in engendering masculinity. At the same time, too, the devaluation of women's lives has taken on many new forms—and not just in India. The issue of the sharp decline in Child Sex Ratios over the nineties due to sex-selective abortions (SSA) has brought this sharply to focus. But while attention is focused on this important issue, it is also important to link this phenomenon to broader forces and ideologies, and indeed policies that engender masculinity. Thus it is often not adequately recognised that the withdrawal of the state—from health, education, employment generation and actively combating anti-women values—engenders both the feminisation of poverty and the shrouding and enfoldment of women, sacrificing them on the altar of the family. As is well known, all religious fundamentalisms write their writs on the bodies of women, becoming particularly acute as they play out the politics of identity. Thus since the 1990s we have seen, in India as in many other parts of the globe, a sharp increase in violent crimes against women. We also recorded a steep rise in violence especially against dalit women (Human Rights Watch 1999).[45] We have also witnessed a significant increase in so-called honour killings, especially in the same areas of north and west India that have also seen an increase of SSA (Chowdhry 2000).[46] The same areas too have witnessed the rebirth, or revitalization, of 'caste panchayats' that have been passing extra-judicial judgements against women, and indeed men, allegedly transgressing the boundaries of caste. A sharp increase in dowry deaths—or more precisely dowry murders—has also been documented in these regions. As Chowdhury has revealed in her study, in all these cases, it is almost impossible to obtain state action (*ibid*).[47] Indeed, new forms of dowry, new forms of crass commercialism, and the disappearance of girl children, appear to go together, as patriarchy and what could be called *karva chauth* capitalism intersect, along with the increasing commodification of women. Some of these areas have also seen the emergence of 'importation' of women for marriage. Some patterns of 'across-region marriages' have emerged: Haryanvi men marrying Assamese women, men in UP importing brides from West Bengal, and men in Rajasthan importing brides from Andhra Pradesh and Tamil Nadu (Kaur 2004).[48] Extreme poverty among groups giving away daughters, along with the low sex ratio in groups importing such brides are seen as crucial factors explaining the increase of such marriages over the last decade or so. In Haryana, where it is reported that girls are brought in from as far away as Orissa and Bangladesh, such girls are apparently referred to as 'lesser wives' (Sangwan 2005).[49] The lesser wives, it is reported, are sometimes 'married' to more than one 'lesser husband', who due to relative poverty and lack of brides, cannot obtain a bride of his caste. Thus we witness the emergence of new forms of sex slavery, along with polyandry, which apparently claims the sanctity of tradition.

The policy initiatives leading to the decline of the state, the rise in fundamentalisms, and the rise in anti-feminisms are all related. All serve to marginalize the concerns of women's health and the health of the poor and otherwise marginalized. The focus on population then serves as a red herring.

NOTES

1. National Planning Committee, Report of the Sub-Committee on National Health, Vora, Bombay, 1948.
2. *Ibid.*
3. NPC, Report of the Sub-Committee on Population, Vora, Bombay, 1948.
4. Chatterjee, Nilanjana and Riley, Nancy E, 'Planning an Indian Modernity: The Gendered Politics of Fertility Control', *Signs, Journal of Women in Culture and Society*, Vol 26, no.3, 2001.
5. Zachariah, Benjamin, 'Uses of Scientific Argument: The Case of 'Development' in India, C.1930 -1950', *Economic and Political Weekly*, Vol.XXXVI, No.39, 2001.
6. Srinivasan, K, Regulating Reproduction in India's Population: Efforts, Results and Recommendations, Sage, New Delhi, 1995.
7. Gandhi M. K., The Collected Works of Mahatma Gandhi,Vol 16, Publications Division, New Delhi, 1920.
8. Srinivasan, *op cit*, 1995.
9. NPC, Report of the Sub Committee on Woman's Role in Planned Economy, Vora, Bombay, 1948.
10. Anandhi, S, 'Reproductive Bodies and Regulated Sexuality: Birth Control Debates in Early Twentieth Century Tamil Nadu' in John Mary E. and Nair Janaki (eds), *A Question of Silence?: The Sexual Economies of Modern India*, Kali for Women, New Delhi, 2000.
11. Rao, Mohan, Population Control to From Reproductive Health: Malthusian Arithmetic, Sage, New Delhi, 2004.
12. Venkatesan, J, 'Two Child Norm Upheld', *The Hindu*, 31st July 2003.
13. Sarkar, Lotika and Ramanathan, Usha, 'Collateral Concerns', *Seminar*, 511, 2002.
14. PTI, 'SC notice to Centre, states on 2-kid norm', *The Indian Express*, 1st March, 2005. This report states that a Bench comprising Chief Justice R.C. Lahoti and Justice D.M.Adhikari issued notices to Haryana, Rajasthan, Madhya Pradesh, Orissa, Andhra Pradesh and Himachal Pradesh, in addition to the Centre. It goes on to say that this notice assumes particular significance "as the Centre was proposing to drop the 2-child norm arguing that coercive methods would not be fruitful in achieving population goals."
15. Hartmann, Betsy, Reproductive Rights and Wrongs: The Global Politics of Population Control, South End Press, Mass, 1995.
16. Lok Sabha Secretariat, The Population Stabilisation Bill, 1999, (Dr. V. Saroja, M.P.), New Delhi, 1999.
17. Lok Sabha Secretariat, The Population Control Bill, 2000, (Mr. U.V. Krishnam Raju, M.P.), New Delhi, 2000.
18. Lok Sabha Secretariat, The Bachelors' Allowance Bill, 2000, (Mr. Chandrakant Khaire, M.P.), New Delhi, 2000.
19. Lok Sabha Secretariat, The Population Control Bill, 2000, (Mr. Y.S. Vivekananda Reddy, M.P.), New Delhi, 2000.
20. Lok Sabha Secretariat, The Population Control and Family Welfare Bill, 1999, (Mr. Sushil Kumar Shinde, M.P.), New Delhi, 1999.
21. Government of Uttar Pradesh, State Law Commission (2002), The Uttar Pradesh Population Control Bill, 2002, Lucknow.
22. Measham Anthony R. and Heaver Richard A, India's Family Welfare

Programme: Towards a Reproductive and Child Health Approach, World Bank, Washington DC, 1995.
23. Rao Mohan, 'Flip Flops on Population Policy' in Rao Mohan (ed), *The Unheard Scream: Reproductive Health and Women's Lives in India*, Zubaan, New Delhi, 2004.
24. Sengupta, Amit, 'The World Bank's Reproductive and Child Health Approach: New Wine in Old Bottles', in Rao Mohan (ed), *Reproductive Health in India's Primary Healthcare*, CSMCH, New Delhi, 1998.
25. 'NGOs, health groups oppose law denying water', *The Hindu*, Wednesday, 13th April 2005.
26. Sharma, Aman, 'Sterilisation-for-gun Backfires for U.P. Govt', *The Indian Express*, 28th August, 2004.
27. Kurup, Saira, 'IMA Bitten by China's One-Child Norm', *The Times of India*, 24th April, New Delhi, 2005.
28. 'Bill to Curb Population on Anvil: Sushma', *The Hindustan Times*, 10th April 2003.
29. Misra Rajiv, Chatterjee Rachel and Rao Sujatha, India Health Report, Oxford University Press, New Delhi, 2003.
30. Qadeer Imrana, 'Reproductive Health: A Public Health Perspective', *Economic and Political Weekly*, Vol.XXX, No.41, 1998.
31. IIPS, National Family Health Survey 1998-99, Mumbai, 2000.
32. Menon Shreelatha, 'The State of the Art Cycle Pumps', in Rao Mohan (ed), *Reproductive Health and Women's Lives in India*, Kali for Women, New Delhi (forthcoming), 2004.
33. van Hollen Cecilia, Birth on the Threshold, Zubaan/Kali for Women, New Delhi, 2001.
34. Jaffery Patricia and Jeffery Roger, Confronting Saffron Demography: Religion, Fertility and Women's Status in India, Three Essays Collective, New Delhi, 2006.
35. Government of India, Planning Commission (Undated), Ninth Five Year Plan 1997-2002, New Delhi.
36. Baru Rama, Private Health in India: Social Chracteristics and Trends, Sage, New Delhi, 1998.
37. Krishnan T.N, 'Access to Health and the Burden of Treatment: An Inter-State Comparison', in Rao Mohan (ed), *Disinvesting in Health: The World Bank Prescriptions for Health*, Sage, New Delhi, 1999.
38. Baru Rama V, and Sadhana G, 'Resurgence of Communicable Diseases; Gastroenteritis Epidemics in Andhra Pradesh', *Economic and Political Weekly*, Vol.XXXV, No.40, 2000.
39. Shariff, *op cit, 1999*.
40. Sengupta Amit, 'Economic Reforms, Health and Pharmaceuticals', *Economic and Political Weekly*, Vol.XXXI, No 48, 1996.
41. Sen Gita, Iyer Aditi and George Asha, 'Class, Gender and Health Equity: Lessons from Liberalizing India' in Sen Gita, George Asha and Ostlin Piroska (eds), *Engendering International Health*, MIT Press, Massachusetts, 2002.
42. *Ibid.*
43. Government of India, Ministry of Health and Family Welfare, *National Health Policy*, New Delhi, 2002.
44. Government of India, Ministry of Statistics and Programme Implementation,

Note on Morbidity and Treatment of Ailmets: NSS 52nd Round (July 1995-June 1996), *Sarvekshana*, Vol.XXIII, No.3, January-March, 2000.

45. Human Rights Watch, Broken People: Caste Violence Against India's 'Untouchables', Books for Change, Bangalore, 1999.
46. Chowdhry Prem, 'Enforcing Cultural Codes: Gender and Violence in Northern India' in John Mary E and Nair Janaki (eds), *A Question of Silence? The Sexual Economies of Modern India*, Kali for Women, New Delhi, 2000.
47. *Ibid.*
48. Kaur Ravinder, 'Across Region Marriages: Poverty, Female Migration and the Sex Ratio', *Economic and Political Weekly*, Vol.39, No.25, 2004.
49. Sangwan, 'Jagmati, Movement Experiences from Haryana', Paper presented at the Silver Jubilee Seminar of the CWDS, Globalisation and the Women's Movement in India, 20th-22nd January, New Delhi, 2005.

9

Pre-conception and Pre-natal Diagnostic Techniques Act 1994: Its Need, Features and Implementation Status

Rattan Chand

1. Introduction

Preference for sons has existed traditionally in India due to various socio-economic, religious and cultural factors like security in old age, carrying forward the name of family and business, performing of religious rites etc. The practice of dowry and daughters being viewed as *paraya dhan* (to be married and sent away) are yet other reasons why sons are preferred to daughters. This obsessive preference for sons, coupled with discrimination against women have, historically, spawned practices like female foeticide, bride burning and sati; and the neglect of girl child in terms of nutrition, education, healthcare etc. Hence, unnatural elimination of girls and women has been going on, leading to adverse sex ratio in India. Various methods were found to eliminate the girl child after her birth like starving her, crushing her under the bed, or giving poison etc. While such practices prevailed, there were also valiant efforts at fighting them by social reformers and hence sex ratio decline has been kept under leash.

Anthropologists and demographers have argued that both infanticide and selective infant and child mortality are means by which parents traditionally attempted to determine or manage the sex composition of their families (Miller 1981; Hausfaster and Hardy 1984). It is the gender composition that is increasingly identified as a key factor in determining the birth and survival of additional children. In the past, gender composition was an important chance factor in the iterative process of family planning. Now, however, parents are able to exercise greater control over the gender composition of their families in addition to the number and spacing of their children through the use of modern technologies like amniocentesis and ultrasound. The emerging trend of having preference for a small family of one son and one daughter and easy availability of sex determination and sex selection may be proving to be catalyst in the process.

2. Magnitude of the Problem

2.1 Decline in Child Sex Ratio

The Child Sex Ratio[1] (CSR) for the age group 0-6 years has declined at an alarming rate in majority of the States/UTs and districts during 1991-2001. At the all-India level, the Child Sex Ratio has declined from 945 in 1991 to 927 in 2001 showing a decline of 18 points. Results from the two rounds of National Family Health Surveys (NFHS) conducted by the International Institute for Population Sciences, Mumbai, also show that the sex ratio at birth has declined from 951 in 1992-93 to 935 in 1998-99 (Retherford and Roy 2003). The CSR has declined from 976 in 1961 to 927 in 2001.

Further, the census data showed that out of the total of 34 States/UTs for which comparative data for 1991 and 2001 is available, 30 states/UTs have shown a decline in the Child Sex Ratio during 1991-2001. Ten states have shown a decline of 30 points or more (Table 1). The four states that have shown an increase in Child Sex Ratio during 1991-2001 are Chattisgarh (1 point), Kerala (2 points), Pondicherry (4 points) and Lakshadweep (18 points).

The comparative data for 1991 and 2001 census is available for 579 districts in the country. The Child Sex Ratio has declined in 476 districts (82 per cent) during 1991-2001 (Table 2). The Child Sex Ratio has, however, remained unchanged in 7 districts and increased in 96 districts. In 60 districts, the Child Sex Ratio has declined by more than 50 points. In one district each in Himachal Pradesh, Punjab

Table 1: Decline in Child Sex Ratio (CSR) in various States/UTs

Decline in points	Number of States*/UTs	States/UTs (decline in CSR)
(1)	(2)	(3)
50 or more	4	Punjab (77), Haryana (60), Himachal Pradesh (55), Chandigarh (54)
30-50	6	Delhi (47), Gujarat (45), Uttranchal (40), D & N Haveli (34), Maharashtra (33), Daman & Diu (32)
20-29	2	Nagaland (29), Goa (26)
10-19	11	Arunachal Pradesh (18), Manipur (17), A & N Islands (16), Andhra Pradesh (14), Jharkhand (14), Karnataka (14), Orissa (14), Meghalaya (13), Bihar (11), Uttar Pradesh (11), Assam (10)
1-9	7	Madhya Pradesh (9), Rajasthan (7), West Bengal (7), Tamil Nadu (6), Mizoram (5), Sikkim (2), Tripura (1)

*excluding J & K.

and Haryana, it has declined by more than 100 points. These are respectively Kangra, Fatehgarh Saheb and Ambala. Majority of the districts have shown decline in almost all states/UTs. The districts of Himachal Pradesh, Punjab, Haryana, Uttaranchal, Delhi, Gujarat and Maharashtra have shown a relatively higher decline in Child Sex Ratio (Table 2).

2.2 States/UTs in Different Ranges of Child Sex Ratio

In 1991, there was not a single state with Child Sex Ratio of less than 850 whereas three states have entered this group in 2001 (Table 3). These are Punjab (798), Haryana (819) and Chandigarh (845). Three states that have child sex ratio between 850-899 are Delhi (868), Gujarat (883) and Himachal Pradesh (896).

Further, there was not a single district in 1991 with Child Sex Ratio of less than 800 (Table 3). In 2001, there are 14 such districts. Among these 14 districts, nine are from Punjab and five from Haryana. Among the ten districts that have the lowest CSR, seven are from Punjab and three from Haryana. These are Fatehgarh Sahib (766), Kurukshetra (771), Patiala (777), Ambala (782), Mansa (782), Kapurthala (785), Bathinda (785), Sangrur (786), Sonipat (788) and Gurdaspur (789).

Table 2: Distribution of Districts by Decline in Child Sex Ratio (CSR)

State/UT	Range of decline in CSR and number of districts						No change	Increase	Total dist.
	100-150	50-100	30-50	20-30	10-20	1-10			
India	**3**	**57**	**79**	**79**	**121**	**137**	**7**	**96**	**579**
1. J & K*	-	-	-	-	-	-	-	-	-
2. Himachal Pradesh	1	4	2	1	1	1	-	2	12
3. Punjab	1	15	1	-	-	-	-	-	17
4. Chandigarh	-	1	-	-	-	-	-	-	1
5. Uttaranchal	-	3	5	3	2	-	-	-	13
6. Haryana	1	12	6	-	-	-	-	-	19
7. Delhi	-	4	3	2	-	-	-	-	9
8. Rajasthan	-	-	2	4	8	6	3	9	32
9. Uttar Pradesh	-	1	10	10	9	19	2	19	70
10. Bihar	-	1	3	5	11	10	-	7	37
11. Sikkim	-	-	1	-	-	-	-	3	4
12. Arunachal Pradesh	-	1	4	1	2	3	-	2	13
13. Nagaland	-	1	2	2	2	1	-	-	8
14. Manipur	-	-	2	-	4	1	-	2	9
15. Mizoram	-	-	1	1	1	3	-	2	8
16. Tripura	-	-	-	-	-	2	-	2	4
17. Meghalaya	-	-	1	3	1	-	-	2	7
18. Assam	-	1	1	2	8	8	1	2	23
19. West Bengal	-	-	-	2	4	11	-	1	18
20. Jharkhand	-	-	2	2	9	4	-	1	18

21.	Orissa	-	-	5	5	11	7	1	1	30
22.	Chhattisgarh	-	-	-	-	8	5	-	3	16
23.	Madhya Pradesh	-	-	2	5	11	17	-	10	45
24.	Gujarat	-	6	12	3	3	1	-	-	25
25.	Daman & Diu	-	1	-	-	-	-	-	1	2
26.	D & N Haveli	-	-	1	-	-	-	-	-	1
27.	Maharashtra	-	5	11	10	3	5	-	1	35
28.	Andhra Pradesh	-	-	-	6	12	3	-	2	23
29.	Karnataka	-	-	1	7	5	11	-	3	27
30.	Goa	-	-	-	2	-	-	-	-	2
31.	Lakshadweep	-	-	-	-	-	-	-	1	1
32.	Kerala	-	-	-	-	-	5	-	9	14
33.	Tamil Nadu	-	-	1	2	6	14	-	7	30
34.	Pondicherry	-	1	-	-	-	-	-	3	4
35.	A & N Islands	-	-	-	1	-	-	-	1	2

* Figures unavailable as census not conducted during 1991.

Table 3: Number of States/UTs and Districts in different ranges of Child Sex Ratio in 1991 and 2001

Range of Child Sex Ratio	Number of States		Number of Districts	
	1991*	2001	1991*	2001
Less than 800	-	1	-	14
800-849	-	2	1	31
850-899	3	3	67	71
900-949	7	9	184	212
950-999	22	19	306	246
1000 or more	1	-	21	5
All	33	34	579	579

*excluding J & K where census 1991 was not conducted.

In 31 districts, the Child Sex Ratio was in the range of 800 - 849, in 2001. Of these, 12 districts are from Haryana, eight are from Punjab, four from Gujarat, two each from Himachal Pradesh and Madhya Pradesh, and one each from Chandigarh, Delhi and Maharashtra.

Further, the Child Sex Ratio is comparatively lower in the affluent regions of Punjab, Himachal Pradesh, Haryana, Delhi, Chandigarh and Gujarat. State/UT-wise position of sex-ratio is shown in Annexure-I.

3. Response of the Government and the Civil Society

The declining sex ratio and the use of pre-natal diagnostic techniques had drawn attention of the activists ever since these techniques were introduced in India in 1970s primarily for the determination of genetic abnormalities. However, subsequently these techniques were widely misused to determine the sex of the foetus and subsequent abortions if the foetus was found to be female (Jeffery, Jeffery and Lyon 1984). An indirect estimate using the data from two rounds of National Family Health Surveys indicates more than 100, 000 sex selective abortions in India every year (Arnold, Kishore and Roy 2002). The evidence of substantial sex-selective abortions in states such as Punjab, Haryana, Delhi and Maharashtra was found to be consistent with the high use of ultrasound and amniocentesis (Retherford and Roy 2003). Due to relentless efforts of activists, a law to prevent sex determination was passed in Maharashtra known as Maharashtra Regulation of Pre-natal Diagnostic Techniques Act

1988. Finally after intense public debate all over India, the Parliament enacted the Pre-natal Diagnostic Techniques (Regulation and Prevention of Misuse) Act, 1994 in order to check the practice of sex determination and to prevent female foeticide. The Act was brought into operation from 1st January, 1996 by the Ministry of Health and Family Welfare. The Pre-natal Diagnostic Techniques Act, 1994 has since been amended to make it more comprehensive. The amended Act and Rules came into force with effect from 14.2.2003 and the PNDT Act has been renamed as Pre-conception and Pre-Natal Diagnostic Techniques (Prohibition of Sex Selection) Act, 1994 (PNDT Act).

3.1 Objectives of PNDT Act

The PNDT Act has twofold objectives:

- The prohibition of sex selection, before or after conception. The purpose is to prevent misuse of such techniques for sex determination that could eventually lead to elimination of the female foetus and thereby create a gender imbalanced society
- The regulation of prenatal diagnostic techniques. It regulates, though does not deny, use of pre-natal diagnostic techniques, such as ultrasound, for the purpose of detecting genetic abnormalities or other sex linked disorders in the foetus (MOHFW 2003).

3.2 Prohibitions and regulations under the Act

- All units providing genetic counselling or providing pre-natal diagnostic techniques must be registered under the Act.
- Sex selection and sex determination for non-medical reasons are prohibited under the Act.
- No person conducting pre-natal diagnostic procedures shall communicate the sex of the foetus by words, signs or in any other form to the pregnant woman or any other person associated with her.
- Pre-natal diagnostic techniques can be conducted only for the purposes mentioned in the Act.
- All units conducting pre-natal diagnostic techniques must prominently display a notice in English and in local language that 'Sex determination of foetus is prohibited under the law'.

- Doctors or clinics advertising sex selection in any form are liable for punishment.
- No manufacturer shall sell ultrasound machines to a unit that is not registered under the Act.

3.3 Who All are Liable under the Act?

- Every person in charge of and responsible for the conduct of business of the unit providing pre-natal diagnostic techniques.
- Persons who perform the tests.
- Mediator who is responsible for advising pregnant women to the unit conducting determination of sex/sex selection.
- Husband/relatives of the pregnant women.
- The pregnant women herself is considered innocent under the Act, unless and until proved otherwise.
- Persons/units advertising about sex selection in any form.

3.4 Inspections/Investigations Against any Violation

Appropriate authorities have been vested with the power of conducting search and seizure operations as part of their investigative powers. Investigations can be initiated based on their own (*suo moto*) belief that a breach of provisions of the Act has taken place or on a complaint filed before them. At the time of conducting investigations, all clinics are obliged to afford all reasonable facilities for inspection of the place, personnel, equipment, and records maintained.

3.5 Penalties under the Act

For breach of any of the provisions of the Act by any of the service providers or their employees, he/she may be imprisoned up to three years and fined up to 10,000 rupees. For any subsequent offences, he/she may be imprisoned up to five years and fined up to 50,000 rupees. The name of the registered medical practitioner is reported by the appropriate authority to the state medical council concerned for taking necessary action including suspension of the registration if the charges are framed by the court and till the case is disposed off and on conviction for removal of his name from the register of the Council for a period of five years for the first offence and permanently for the subsequent offence. Similarly the persons seeking sex selection or seeking to know the sex of the foetus can be imprisoned up to five years and fined up to 100,000 rupees.

4. How can the Medical Community Help in Implementation of the PC and PNDT Act?

PC and PNDT Act demand ethical medical practice so that the medical technology which is for the benefit of the masses is not misused for sex determination or sex selection. The medical community can help in implementation of the Act in the following ways:

- Counsel their patients and families about the importance of girl child and the adverse impact of the skewed sex ratio on the society.
- Desist from conducting sex selection/sex determination. If medical community says no to sex selection, it will not happen.
- To impress upon their colleagues not to practise sex selection/ determination and report about the erring colleagues to the concerned Appropriate Authorities.
- Get registered with the appropriate authority in the area if the unit uses any of the pre-natal diagnostic techniques.
- A notice should be displayed by the units conducting pre-natal diagnostic techniques that 'Disclosure of the sex of the foetus is prohibited under the law'.
- Maintain all records properly and follow the standards prescribed regarding qualified persons and space under the Act.

5. Implementation Status of the PC and PNDT Act

The implementation of the Act rests with the states/UTs through the appropriate authorities constituted at state, district and sub-district level. The Act provides for three kinds of implementing bodies, viz. policy making bodies, appropriate authorities and advisory committees.

5.1 Policy Making Bodies

The Central and State Supervisory Boards are the policy making bodies constituted under the Act. The Central Supervisory Board is headed by the Union Minister for Health and Family Welfare, whereas the State Supervisory Board is headed by the Minister in charge of Health and Family Welfare of the concerned state. These boards have government representatives, non-official members from amongst medical geneticists, gynaecologists and obstetricians, paediatricians, social scientists, women activists and women Members of Parliament. These bodies are primarily responsible for advising the central and state governments on policy matters. They are also responsible for overseeing the performance of various bodies constituted under the Act and creating awareness on the issue of sex selection and sex selective abortions.

5.2 Appropriate Authorities (AAs)

These are the main implementing authorities for enforcement of the PC and PNDT Act. These authorities are appointed at the state, district and sub-district level. At the state level, it is a three-member body with Director/Joint Director, Family Welfare, representative of an eminent women organization and an officer of law department as members. At the district and sub-district levels, Chief Medical Officer and Medical Officer in charge of sub-district are the Appropriate Authorities. All states have constituted state level/ district level Appropriate Authorities and Advisory Committees.

The main functions of the AAs are:

- Granting, rejecting, suspending, cancelling registrations.
- Conducting inspections and investigations.
- Creating public awareness.
- Preparing quarterly reports on implementation of the Act and sending these to the higher authorities.
- Recommending changes in the Act and Rules for better implementation.

5.3 Advisory Committees

Each appropriate authority is aided and advised by the advisory committee constituted for it. This committee consists of social workers and experts in medicine, law, and communication/ information.

5.4 Registration of Units

All units providing pre-natal diagnostic technique services are required to be registered under the Act. Although the Act was passed in 1994, it could not be effectively implemented during the initial years after its enactment. Even in the year 1998, all states had not established implementing authorities required under the Act. The results of Census 2001 indicated an alarming decline in Child Sex Ratio. A public interest litigation (PIL) was filed in the Supreme Court in the year 1998 with the objective to implement the law and to include the pre-conception sex selection techniques under the ambit of the law. The PIL was finally disposed off on 10.9.2003. The registration of bodies gained momentum after 2001. As per the reports received up to 28.02.2006 from various States/UTs, 28027 bodies using ultrasound machines, image scanners etc. have been registered. Majority of the bodies were registered in the year 2001-02 (Figure 1).

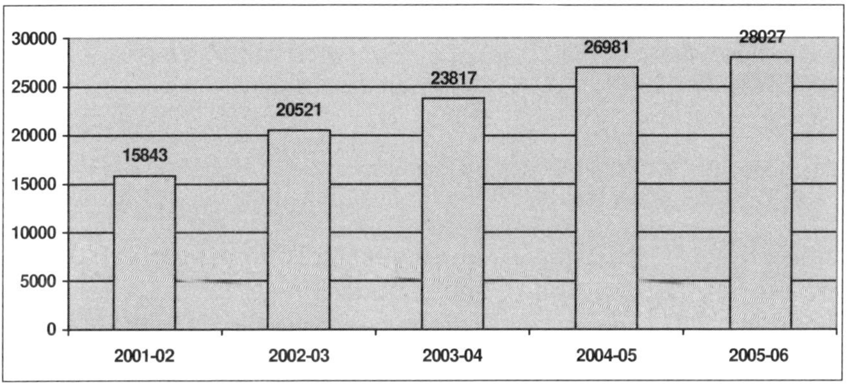

Figure 1: Commulative Number of Bodies Registered

5.5 Types of Bodies Registered

Depending upon the kind of services provided, units can be registered as genetic counselling centres, genetic clinics, and genetic laboratories. Clinics conducting ultrasound/imaging tests for the purpose other than pre-natal diagnostic care have to be registered as ultrasound clinics or imaging centres, as applicable. Majority of the registered bodies (16454 or 58.7 per cent of the total) belong to the category of ultrasound clinics/imaging centres (Figure 2).

5.6 Types of Violations Encountered

As per reports received up to 31.3.2005, 303 cases are being tried in various courts for various violations of the law. These violations relate to non-registration, non-maintenance of accounts, communication of sex of foetus, advertisements about pre-

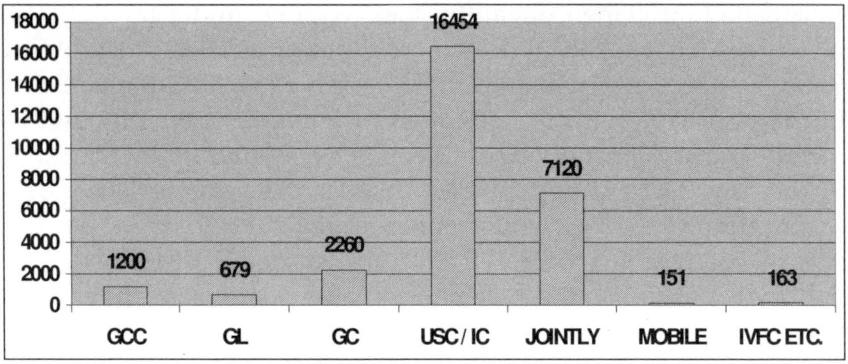

Figure 2: Registration by Type of Unit

Note: GCC—Genetic Counselling Centres.
GL—Genetic Laboratories.
GC—Genetic Clinics.
USC/IC—Ultrasound Clinics/Imaging Centres.
Jointly—JAGCC/GL/GC—Jointly as Genetic Counselling Centres/Gen. Labs./Gen. Clinics.
Mobile—MC(V)—Mobile Clinics (Vehicles).
IVF etc.—Other bodies/IVF Centres/Infertility Centres.

conception/pre-natal facility etc (Figure 3). Though most of the cases are on non-registration of the centre/clinics, 37 cases relate to determination and disclosure of the sex of the foetus in the States of Haryana (12), Karnataka (1), Maharashtra (8), Punjab, Tamil Nadu (1) (13) and Uttaranchal (2). Twenty-eight cases also exist against

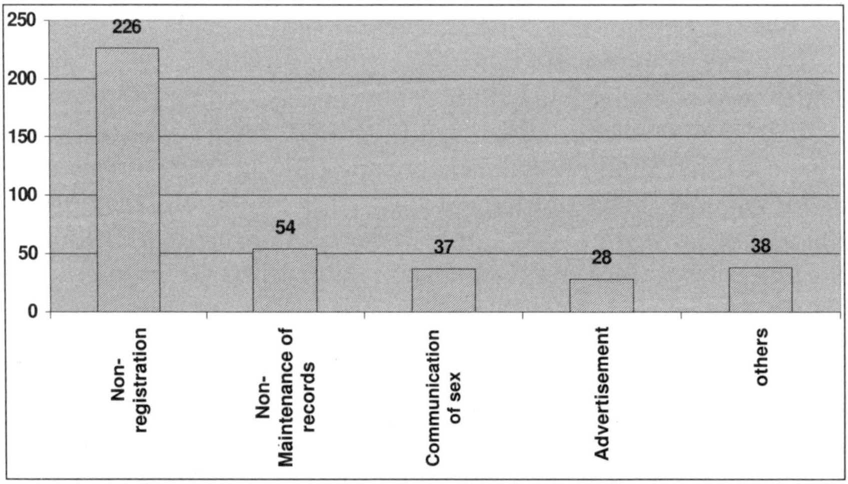

Figure 3: Existing Court Cases by Type of Violation

people who have given advertisement about facilities of pre-conception/pre-natal sex selection in the states of Gujarat (3), Haryana (5), Madhya Pradesh (4), Maharashtra (6), Rajasthan (1), Tamil Nadu (1), Uttaranchal (1), Uttar Pradesh (1) and Delhi (6). Two hundred and forty-two cases have already been disposed off. State governments are requested from time to time to take effective measures for speedy disposal of ongoing cases.

5.7 Other Steps Taken by the Government

It is recognized by the government that mere legislation is not enough to deal with this problem that has roots in social behaviour and prejudices. Various activities have been undertaken to create awareness against the practice of pre-natal determination of sex and female foeticide which include:

- Advertisements through radio, television, and print media.
- Workshops and seminars through NGOs at state/regional/district/block levels.
- Seeking cooperation from elected representatives, religious leaders, as well as medical fraternity.
- Training of judiciary.
- Launching of the 'Save the Girl Child' campaign with a view to lessening preference for sons by highlighting achievements of young girls.
- Disseminating data through maps. A booklet titled 'Missing', showing maps and posters exhibiting areas of adverse child sex ratio in India has been brought out.
- Handbook on PNDT Act, 1994 and Amendments has been published. The Act and Rules have been placed in the website of the Ministry of Health and Family welfare.
- Publishing of the Act and Rules in the Journal of Indian Medical Association with appeal from the Secretary, Ministry of Health and Family Welfare to the medical community to restrain from sex determination and sex selection.

5.7.1 National Inspection and Monitoring Committee

A National Inspection and Monitoring Committee has been constituted on the directions of the Supreme Court at the Centre to take stock of the ground realities by field visits to the problem States. The reports of the visits are placed in the meetings of the Central

Supervisory Board under the chairmanship of the Union Minister of Health and Family Welfare. The Committee has already visited a number of districts in the states of Haryana, Punjab, Gujarat, Rajasthan, Maharashtra, Uttar Pradesh, Uttaranchal and Tamil Nadu, Union Territory of Chandigarh and NCT of Delhi. The committee has since been reconstituted in March 2005 and representatives from National Commission for Women, Indian Council for Medical Research and Department of Women and Child Development have also been included in the committee.

5.7.2 National Support and Monitoring Cell

The success of implementation of the PC & PNDT Act depends upon identifying the wrongdoers and catching them red-handed. However, only 37 cases of sex determination and communication have been booked so far at the all-India level. A National Support and Monitoring Cell is being constituted on a pilot basis to strengthen the capabilities of the appropriate authorities of problem states like Punjab, Haryana, Gujarat and Delhi in identifying the wrongdoers and in apprehending them.

5.7.3 Training of Judiciary

With a view to sensitise the judiciary, services of the National Judicial Academy, Bhopal was being taken during 2005-06. The National Judicial Academy would first provide training to trainers from the state judicial academies that in turn will provide training to the judiciary in the area under their jurisdiction.

5.7.4 Frequently Asked Questions

The Ministry of Health and Family Welfare, in collaboration with the United Nations Population Fund (UNFPA), are developing 'Frequently Asked Questions' about the PC & PNDT Act which will be useful to lay people, medical communities and appropriate authorities in understanding the provisions of the Act for better implementation.

6. Conclusions

Declining child sex ratio is a matter of grave concern and to check this, the government has been enforcing the Pre-conception and Prenatal Diagnostic Techniques Act since 1996. The machinery for implementation of the PNDT Act has been put in place in the country and the units providing PNDT services have been registered. Awareness about the law has also been created. However, it is difficult to catch the wrong doers as both the service seekers and service providers are in league and mostly there is no complainant. Although there are over 380 cases in various courts, only 38 cases relate to sex determination. The establishment of the Support and Monitoring Cell is likely to help in strengthening the capabilities of the appropriate authorities in identifying and apprehending the wrongdoers. The trend in declining child sex ratio can be arrested with the joint efforts of the government and civil society.

NOTE

1. Child Sex Ratio is defined as number of girls per 1000 boys in the age group of 0-6 years.

REFERENCES

Arnold Fred, Kishore Sunita, and Roy T.K., 'Sex Selective Abortions in India', *Population and Development Review*, Vol. 28 (4), 2002.

GOI, Handbook on PNDT Act, 1994 and Amendments (revised edition), Department of Family Welfare, Government of India, February 2003.

Hausfater and Hrdy Blaffer (eds), Infanticide: Comparative and Evolutionary Perspectives, New York, 1984.

Jeffery Roger, Jeffery Patricia and Lyon Andrew, 'Female Infanticide and Amniocentesis', *Social Sciences and Medicine*, 19: pp 1201-12, 1984.

Lawyers Collective, Pre-conception & Pre-natal Diagnostic Techniques Act, A Users Guide to the Law, The Lawyers Collective, Women's Rights Initiative, Universal Law Publishing Co, 2004.

MOHFW, 'Missing ... Mapping the Adverse Child Sex Ratio in India', Ministry of Health and Family Welfare, Registrar-General of India and United Nations Population Fund, November, 2003.

Miller B.D., The Endangered Sex, Cornell University Press, Ithaca, New York, 1981.

Population Stabilization and Sustainable Development, Population Foundation of India, New Delhi.

Retherford R.D. and Roy T.K., 'Factors Affecting Sex Selective Abortions in India and 17 Major States', National Family Health Survey Report, No. 21, Mumbai, IIPS and Hawaii, East-West Centre, 2003.

ANNEXURE-I

State/UT-wise Sex ratio and Child Sex Ratio (0-6 years) during 1991 & 2001

India and State/ Union territory*	Sex ratio		Child Sex Ratio (0-6 years)		
	1991	2001	1991	2001	Change
(1)	(2)	(3)	(4)	(5)	(6)
INDIA	**927**	**933**	**945**	**927**	18
Jammu & Kashmir	896	892	NA	941	NA
Himachal Pradesh	**976**	**968**	**951**	**896**	55
Punjab	**882**	**876**	**875**	**798**	77
Chandigarh *	790	777	899	845	54
Uttaranchal	936	962	948	908	40
Haryana	**865**	**861**	**879**	**819**	60
Delhi *	827	821	915	868	47
Rajasthan	910	921	916	909	7
Uttar Pradesh	876	898	927	916	11
Bihar	907	919	953	942	11
Sikkim	878	875	965	963	2
Arunachal Pradesh	859	893	982	964	18
Nagaland	886	900	993	964	29
Manipur	958	978	974	957	17
Mizoram	921	935	969	964	5
Tripura	945	948	967	966	1
Meghalaya	955	972	986	973	13
Assam	923	935	975	965	10
West Bengal	917	934	967	960	7
Jharkhand	922	941	979	965	14
Orissa	971	972	967	953	14
Chhattisgarh	985	989	974	975	-1
Madhya Pradesh	912	919	941	932	9
Gujarat	934	920	928	883	45
Daman & Diu*	969	710	958	926	32
Dadra & Nagar Haveli*	952	812	1013	979	34
Maharashtra	934	922	946	913	33
Andhra Pradesh	972	978	975	961	14
Karnataka	960	965	960	946	14
Goa	967	961	964	938	26
Lakshadweep*	943	948	941	959	-18
Kerala	1,036	1,058	958	960	-2
Tamil Nadu	974	987	948	942	6
Pondicherry*	979	1,001	963	967	-4
Andaman & Nicobar Islands*	818	846	973	957	16

*Union Territory.

Source: Census 1991 & 2001, O/O Registrar General of India.

10

Decentralized Governance and Healthcare: Role of Panchayati Raj Institutions

Pradeep Panda

Introduction

In the last two decades, there has been a significant move towards decentralization in most of the developing countries including India. The Constitution of India paved the way for decentralization at the local level with a landmark constitutional reform in 1992—the 73rd and 74th amendments to the Constitution. With these amendments, India's two-tier federal system of a Central Government and state governments became a three-tier system with the inclusion of local governments. Under the tier of state, locally elected bodies are the Panchayati Raj Institutions (PRIs) at the district (zila parishad), block (panchayat samitis), and village (grama panchayat) levels in rural areas, and a similar structure for urban areas comprising municipal corporations and municipal councils (nagar palikas).

There are three important aspects of decentralization—administrative, political and fiscal. For an effective decentralization, the local governments should have the power to make decisions on all the aspects of decentralization. It is fundamental to making governance at the local level more responsive to the felt needs of the large majority of the population, and to effectively reach out to the poor. The decentralized delivery of health, education and infrastructure services to disadvantaged groups and regions are necessary to achieve these goals.

Decentralization is widely perceived to provide a range of potential benefits. Firstly, it is a way of reducing the role of the state by reducing centralized command and control and introducing more inter-governmental competition and checks and balances. Secondly, it is a way to make government more responsive and efficient. Thirdly, the lower levels of governments now have a greater ability to provide public services, e.g. roads, electricity, water supply, health, education etc. Fourthly, decentralization is viewed as a way of diffusing social and political tensions and ensuring local cultural and political autonomy (Bardhan, 2002). However, Bardhan cautions that decentralization, to be effective in service delivery, has to accompany serious attempts to change the existing structures of power within communities and to improve the opportunities for participation and voice and engaged the hitherto disadvantaged in the political process. Unless these reforms are undertaken, local governments may be subject to capture by elites (Bardhan and Mookherjee, 2006).

The evidence about the potential benefits of decentralization in developing countries is mixed. For instance, in order to examine the impact of decentralization on health sector allocative efficiency in Uganda, it was found that local government health planners are allocating declining proportions of their budgets to public goods activities (Akin, Hutchinson and Trrumpf, 2005). A study in South Africa found that the relationships, structures and processes of local governance could limit both the space for women's participation and the policy potential for addressing gender issues (Beall, 2005). An evaluation of the newly suggested structure of local government in Bangladesh reveals that the critical element of autonomy has not been built into the process of decentralization although democracy and participation are often suggested as the normative basis for decentralization (Westergaard and Alam, 1995). A comparative analysis of decentralization in Pakistan, Indonesia and the Philippines suggests that the Philippines programme has attained better performance compared to the other two countries. The author attributes the following factors for the success of decentralization in the Philippines: (a) a broad supervisory institutional structure, (b) substantial international inputs into the development of the legal and regulatory framework, (c) innovative capacity-building exercises and institutions, (d) strong interest in monitoring and evaluation of the devolution programme, (e) provision of sufficient local fiscal autonomy, (f) efforts to streamline local government operation, and (g) efforts to replace input budgeting and legal management with systems driven by performance incentives and targets (Guess, 2005).

Empirical Evidence of the Impact of Decentralization in India

In India too, the impact of decentralization is mixed. Asthana (2003) shows that the benefits of decentralization are not as obvious as the standard theory of fiscal federalism predicts. The author examines the effect of decentralization of provision of drinking water in central India. The study shows that the decentralized provision of water supply under the control of local governments is less efficient as compared to the provision of water supply under state government. Another study by Johnson, Deshinger and Start (2005) compared the more ambitious decentralization agenda of Madhya Pradesh with the somewhat less decentralized Andhra Pradesh. They found that certain forms of poverty reduction empowered the poor in Andhra Pradesh whereas such an impact was not visible in Madhya Pradesh. This discrepancy is explained by the authors as caused by two factors — (a) decentralization in Madhya Pradesh failed to challenge the well-entrenched power of the sarpanches of the village panchayats, (b) the development populism in Andhra Pradesh was successful in reaching to and empowering the poor (e.g., provision of subsidized rice to low-income households and credit to women's self-help groups).

Mahal *et al* (2000), using a village-level data set in India, test the hypothesis that increased decentralization positively influences health and education outcomes, such as school enrolment and infant mortality rate. The study, however, did not find robust results that suggest positive impact of decentralization on outcomes. Another study compared the effects of decentralization in Karnataka (India), Bangladesh, Cote d'Ivoire and Ghana. Karnataka seemed to have performed better compared to the other three countries due to a more effective system of democratic accountability, an established party system and a free press. They found positive effects of decentralization in terms of increased attendance of school teachers, and efficient and quick response to popular pressures by the local governments (Crook and Manor, 1998).

On the basis of data from 265 Village Councils in West Bengal and Rajasthan, a recent study found that the panchayat has effective control over the policy decisions at the local level. Interestingly, women elected as leaders under the reservation policy invest more in public goods more closely linked to women's concerns (e.g. drinking water and roads in West Bengal and drinking water in Rajasthan). However, they invest less in public goods that are more closely linked to men's concerns (e.g. education in West Bengal and roads in Rajasthan) (Chattopadhyay and Duflo, 2004).

In India, with respect to public service delivery in health sector, the Hospital Development Committees of Kerala and the *Rogi Kalyan Samitis* of Madhya Pradesh are good models. However, the nature and degree of decentralization vary between these two states. In Kerala, the hospitals have been transferred to local Panchayati Raj Institutions (PRIs) and the committee is headed by the PRI president/ chairperson. In Rajasthan, a member of the legislative assembly (MLA) is nominated to the society board and PRIs are not recognized as important stakeholders (Sadanandan and Shiv Kumar, 2006). In this paper, we focus on the role of PRIs as the local governance mechanism in the provision of healthcare.

In spite of the existence of political empowerment of PRIs, including representation of backward castes and women, this has not translated into empowerment in other spheres. Moreover, while state governments are expected to transfer the three Fs (functions, funds and functioning), in practice most states have transferred only one F, i.e., functions to the PRIs. The three states where substantial resources are being transferred to PRIs are Kerala, Karnataka and Madhya Pradesh. In Karnataka the allocations are largely to the zila panchayats. Genuine devolution has taken place only in Kerala in the sense of transferring resources and responsibilities to lower levels of government.

Therefore, the present paper focuses on Kerala's decentralized experiment to understand the trajectory of the processes of decentralized development in Kerala, to evaluate the successes and prospects of decentralization for the provision of health services in Kerala, and to draw some lessons from Kerala's experience.

The paper is organized as follows: First, the main features of the

73rd Constitutional Amendment and scopes and functions of the Gram Sabha are discussed; second, key features of Kerala's decentralization and operationalization of decentralized participatory planning are examined; third, Kerala's health sector under decentralization is dealt with; fourth, the impact of decentralized planning on health sector in Kerala is examined by critically reviewing the empirical studies; fifth, the lessons learnt so far and the action taken by the government to overcome some of the constraints are presented; finally, the paper concludes with some recommendations for the sustainability of Kerala's decentralization efforts and possible lessons that could be drawn from Kerala's experience for other states in India.

Features of the 73rd Constitutional Amendment

The 73rd Constitutional Amendment is concerned with the Panchayati Raj Institutions (PRIs). Table 1 presents the features of the 73rd Amendment. According to deSouza (2003) there are four items in the features that could undermine the rural power structure. First, reservation of seats for women, dalits and adivasis in the panchayat, and reservation of chairperson (sarpanch) posts for them is a route for empowerment for these marginalized groups. This gives a voice and a public face to groups that have hitherto been denied these opportunities. Second, institutionalization of decentralized planning is done through the district planning committee (DPC). The DPC is expected to prepare an integrated plan for the district with the participation of people in the planning process, and by implication takes into account the local needs. Third, the creation of state election commission (SEC) and state finance commission (SFC) has broadened the base of the governance structure. The SEC's task is to conduct regular free and fair election without the interference of the state government. The SFC's recommendations could be regarded as the baseline for discussions on the fiscal aspects of decentralized governance.

Fourth, the institutionalization of the village assembly (grama sabha) is to serve as watchdog, checking on the working of the village council (grama panchayat). Table 2 shows the scope and functions of the grama sabha. There is a need to make grama sabha very effective by encouraging participation.

Table 1: Features of the 73rd Constitutional Amendment

1. The centrality of the village assembly (grama sabha), as a deliberate and deciding body, for decentralized governance.
2. A uniform three-tier structure across the country, with the village, block, and district at the appropriate levels. States with population of less than two million have the option of not introducing the intermediate level.
3. Direct election to all seats for all members at all levels. In addition, the chairpersons of the village councils (panchayats) may be made members of the councils (panchayats) at the intermediate level, and chairpersons of block councils (panchayats) at the intermediate level may be members at the district level. Members of Parliament, members of legislative assemblies, and members of legislative councils may also be members of panchayats at the intermediate and district levels.
4. In all the panchayats, seats are reserved for Scheduled Castes (henceforth SCs or dalits) and Scheduled Tribes (henceforth STs or adivasis) in proportion to their population. One-third of the total seats are reserved for women. One-third of the seats reserved for SCs and STs will also be reserved for women.
5. Offices of the chairpersons of the panchayats at all levels will be reserved in favour of SCs and STs in proportion to their population in the state. One-third of the offices of chairpersons of panchayats at all levels will also be reserved for women.
6. The legislature of a state is at liberty to provide the reservation of seats and offices of the chairpersons in panchayats in favour of members of the backward classes.
7. The average panchayat has a uniform five-year term. Elections are to be completed before the expiry of the term. In the event of dissolution, elections will be compulsorily held within six months. The constituted panchayat will serve for the remaining period of the five-year term.
8. It will not be possible to dissolve the existing panchayats by the amendment of any act before its term is ended.
9. A person who is disqualified under any law of the state will not be entitled to become a member of a panchayat.
10. An independent Sate Election Commission to be established for superintendence, direction, and control of the electoral process and preparation of electoral rolls.
11. Devolution of powers and responsibilities by the state in the preparation and implementation of development plans.
12. Setting up of a State Finance Commission once in five years to revise the financial positions of these Panchayati Raj Institutions (PRIs) and to make suitable recommendations to the state on the distribution of funds among panchayats.

Source: deSouza (2003).

Table 2: Scope and Functions of the Grama Sabha

The Grama Sabha is empowered to:

(a) examine annual statements of accounts and audit reports
(b) discuss the report of the preceding year
(c) review programmes of work for the year or any new programme suggested
(d) consider proposals for fresh taxation or for enhancement of existing taxes
(e) select schemes, beneficiaries, and locations
(f) mobilize voluntary labour and contribution-in-kind and cash for the community welfare programmes
(g) render assistance in the implementation of development schemes and rendering services in villages
(h) undertake programmes for adult education and family welfare within the village
(i) promote unity and harmony among all sections of society
(j) consider the budget prepared by the grama panchayat and the future development programmes and plans of the sabha area
(k) consider and scrutinize the existing schemes and all kinds of activities of panchayats
(l) maintain a complete register for all development work undertaken by the grama panchayat or by any other government departments
(m) scrutinize the completed works.

Source: Jain (1997); deSouza (2003).

Decentralized Planning in Kerala

This section provides an overview of the key features of Kerala's decentralization initiative.

Kerala started the decentralization process with a big bang approach, i.e. functions, power and resources (human and financial) were transferred from the state to the local governments simultaneously, without waiting for capacity building and accountability. Kerala followed a campaign approach for participatory local level planning known as 'People's Planning Campaign' to operationalize decentralization. The idea behind this approach was to create a new politics of development at the grassroots level and also a new culture of development that is bottom-up, demand-led and participatory. This approach was helpful to gather support for public action, generated huge demand in the community and helped push the agenda for decentralization. The campaign phase has been completed and the institutionalization phase has begun. There has been continuous support for decentralized planning regardless of the political affiliations of the governments ruling the state at different time periods. The current institutionalization phase continues though very slowly.

Key Features of Kerala's Decentralization

(a) Delineation of function: Prior to decentralization, the government at the district level was responsible for all the development planning activities such as agriculture and allied sectors, irrigation, traditional industries, poverty reduction programmes, education, healthcare, water supply and sanitation, electricity, roads, construction of school buildings, office buildings and anganwadi centres, women and child development, housing and social welfare of the disabled and destitute. After decentralization, almost all these development functions have been transferred to local governments. Table 3 highlights this aspect of the devolution of power to local governments.

Table 3: Devolution of Power to Local Governments

(a) In the health sector: all institutions other than medical colleges and big regional speciality hospitals have been placed under the control of the local governments.

(b) The entire public sanitation and almost the whole of rural water supply scheme are now under the local government's responsibility.

(c) In the education sector: high schools in rural areas have been transferred to the district panchayats and lower primary and upper primary schools to village panchayats; and in urban areas, all schools have been transferred to the urban local bodies.

(d) In the agriculture and allied sectors: the following are now in the domain of the local government functions—Agricultural extension including farmer-oriented support for increasing production and productivity; Watershed management and minor irrigation; Dairy development; Animal husbandry including veterinary care; Inland fisheries.

(e) All the poverty alleviation schemes, including centrally sponsored anti-poverty programmes, are now planned and implemented through the local bodies.

(f) In the field of Social Welfare: barring statutory functions relating to juvenile justice, all the functions are now carried out by local governments. The Integrated Child Development Scheme (ICDS) is fully implemented by village panchayats and urban local bodies. Similarly, care of the disabled has become a local government responsibility to a substantial degree.

(g) The local governments now administer all the welfare pensions.

(h) Connectivity (roads), except highways and major district roads, has become a local government responsibility.

(i) The responsibility for promotion of tiny, cottage and small industries is now mostly with the local governments.

Source: Government of Kerala (2006).

(b) Transfer of human resources: Along with the transfer of development functions, the government transferred institutions, offices and staff to the local governments. The cadre of the staff transferred remained unchanged and the government pays the salaries. The local governments are empowered to have managerial control over the staff. Although transfer of human resources to the local government has not been an easy task, the government could achieve this objective through constant negotiations, training to build trust, amendments of law about code of conduct, norms about staff transfer etc.

(c) Transfer of financial resources: In addition to delineation of functions and transfer of human resources, one-third of the Plan funds are earmarked for local governments and nearly nine-tenths of the Plan funds are given in an untied form to the local governments. In addition, centrally-sponsored and state-sponsored plan schemes that constitute about one-tenth of the Plan grant-in-aid is given to the local governments with clear guidelines about how to spend these state-sponsored schemes. The main features of Kerala's financial devolution to local governments are presented in Table 4.

Table 4: Devolution of Funds to Local Governments

(a) The quantum of Plan funds earmarked for local governments has been unique in the country in the sense of being highest, with the rural local governments getting a 70 to 85 per cent share in accordance with the rural population and the district and block panchayats sharing only the remaining more or less equally.

(b) Around 90 per cent of the Plan funds have been given in a practically untied form to the local governments to prepare and implement their own projects within certain broad policy framework, stipulating that at least 40 per cent of the funds (10 per cent in urban areas) be invested in productive sectors and not more than 30 per cent (50 per cent in urban areas) on roads, and at least 10 per cent be earmarked for gender sensitive schemes. The broad policy framework has also fixed a consensual upper ceiling for subsidies in different categories of schemes.

(c) The entire Plan grants are fully investible (that is, without involving any staff salary or other administrative cost commitments, which normally take away 20 or 25 per cent of the Plan at the state level).

(d) Since the entire Plan grants due to local governments are separately budgeted in a document given as Annexure IV of the State Budget, which is passed by the Legislature, the grants remain non-divertible for other purposes by the executive.

(e) There has been designed a flow of funds procedure, by which the funds flow in four instalments. A local government is expected to spend at least 75 per cent of its allocation during a year, failing which the next year's allotment gets reduced by such shortfall.

Source: Government of Kerala (2006).

Operationalizing Decentralized Participatory Planning

The salient features of People's Planning Campaign are presented below (Isaac and Franke, 2000).

The first stage was 'Needs Identification'. The felt needs of the community were identified through a meeting of the grama sabha/ ward sabha, chaired by an elected representative and coordinated by an official. The methodology adopted to identify felt needs was semi-structured plenary sessions and sub-group sessions dealing with specific developmental issues.

The second stage was 'Situation Analysis'. A situation analysis was conducted based on the felt needs of the community and developmental data collected through primary and secondary sources. The situation analysis was then presented in the form of development reports that described the status in each sector of development with directions for further development.

The third stage was 'Strategy Setting'. Strategy setting was based on a one-day development seminar at the level of local government to discuss the development report. Various stakeholders such as subject experts, elected representatives, nominated sabha members and others, attended the seminar. It provided the over-all directions for setting priorities and strategies of various developmental projects.

The fourth stage was 'Projectisation'. For each development sector at the local government level, a project was prepared that described the objectives, rationale, design and implementation of activities. Various working groups comprising elected representatives, government officials and a non-government subject experts prepared the projects.

The fifth stage was 'Plan Finalization'. The panchayat takes a final decision on the choice of the projects and the annual plan is submitted to the District Planning Committee (DPC) through the Expert Committees.

The sixth stage was 'Plan Vetting'. The Expert Committees at the Block or District level comprising professionals from the government and non-government sectors vet the projects for their technical and financial viability and for conformity with the mandatory government guidelines. These committees can ask for rectification, if any, but are not empowered to change priorities or projects.

The last stage was 'Plan Approval'. Finally, the local government can implement the project after the formal approval from DPC.

The various phases of the planning process during the Ninth Five Year Plan with a built-in gender component at each stage are presented in Table 5.

Table 5: Phases of the Planning Process during Ninth Plan

Phase	Period	Objective	Activities	Gender Component
I. Grama Sabha	Aug. to Oct. 1997	Identify the felt needs of the people	Grama Sabhas in rural areas and ward conventions in urban areas	Special subject group in the Grama Sabhas to discuss gender problems
II. Development Seminar	Oct. to Dec. 1997	Objective assessment of the resources, problems and formulation of local government perspective	Participatory studies: Preparation of development reports, organization of development seminars	Special chapter in development report on gender issues. Special subject group for discussing gender issues in the development seminar
III. Task Forces	Nov. 1997 to March 1998	Preparation of projects	Meeting of task forces	A special task force for women development projects
IV. Elected Bodies	March to June 1998	Formulation of plan at grassroots tiers	Plan formulation meetings of elected representatives	A separate chapter on women's development project. Ten per cent to be set apart for women component plan
V. Voluntary Technical Corps	May to Oct. 1998	Appraisal and approval of plans	Meetings of expert committees	

Source: Government of Kerala (2006).

It may be noted that Kerala has followed good governance practices, capacity building initiatives and an activist facilitator role throughout the implementation process of decentralized planning. Some of the important governance practices in local governments include, (a) accountability, (b) participation, (c) transparency and right to information, (d) IEC campaigns, (e) accreditation of NGOs to act as support agencies for local governments, (f) code of conduct for elected representatives and officials, and (g) Citizen's Charter. As regards capacity building, about 75 key resource persons provide training to about 50 persons on an average from each district. Also, 15 handbooks have been prepared for various sectors including health. It is important to note that the state government has played an activist role throughout the decentralization process to help the local government.

In spite of physical achievements in many sectors of development, the decentralization experiment has generated many challenges that need to be sorted out for enhancing well-being of the disadvantaged groups in Kerala (Table 6).

Table 6: Initial Challenges of Decentralization

(a) No staff increase has been provided for, and exemption made only in a few cases of professionals and highly skilled technical personnel and in special schemes with assistance for staff.

(b) The outliers like Scheduled Tribes are still to gain from decentralization. In a scenario where one section of the poor lives off another section, decentralization has certain inbuilt limitations.

(c) The poorest among the poor need social safety nets particularly for food and health emergencies. This cannot be provided for by local governments.

(d) The management of services, particularly health and education have not been more efficient than before and these services have direct implications for local development especially poverty reduction.

(e) The flow of bank credit into local schemes has been limited resulting more from bankers' reluctance to deal with local governments than from inadequacies of project formulations. This has resulted in higher subsidies.

(f) In a state like Kerala where the number of educated poor is very high there is an inherent limitation in local government action. Linkages with job markets through skill up-gradation or identification of self-employment opportunities or small-scale production activities with assured markets are all functions which can be done better at higher levels.

(g) There is a tendency to spread resources thinly with preference being given to every electoral constituency whenever a development scheme is taken up. Distribution of assets and inputs, not necessarily productive, has been common.

(h) Vertical integration of local level programmes has proved difficult to achieve.

(i) Participatory aspect of planning is often limited to airing of needs and sharing of benefits. There is need for enhancing the quality of participatory planning so that there is a healthy discussion by all sections of the population based on data and norms, generating a prioritized list of development needs.

Source: Vijayanand (2001), quoted in Government of Kerala (2006).

The Government of Kerala has implemented the recommendations of the Second State Finance Commission. Now, resource flow to local governments has increased substantially especially to take care of critical maintenance requirement. However, other recommendations of the finance commission have not yet been operationalized so far that are important to improve the financial base of the local governments.

The Government of Kerala, with 8000 crores rupees earmarked for local governments for the Tenth Plan, has initiated several initiatives during 2004 to strengthen institutionalization of decentralization (Government of Kerala, 2005). These include: (a) a local self-government action plan; (b) a modernizing government programme (MGP); (c) a decentralization support programme, and (d) a project for capacity development for decentralization (Government of Kerala, 2006).

Kerala's Health Sector under Decentralization

Since 1999, local governments manage all the health institutions in Kerala, ranging from Primary Health Centres (PHCs) to District Hospitals. The local governments control and manage all the personnel in these institutions including the District Medical Officer. While the government pays salaries to the health personnel, their recruitment, placement and promotion are the responsibilities of the Health Department. The local governments have complete managerial control over the health personnel including performance monitoring. They have full disciplinary control over the non-gazetted officers, and some disciplinary control over the gazetted health personnel.

Excluding the supply of drugs, all other expenses related to the running of hospitals are transferred to the local governments. The local governments have complete autonomy to prioritize and spend these allocated funds. A senior medical officer under a local government acts as the implementing officer who takes overall responsibility to implement the programmes including record keeping and management of accounts.

As discussed earlier about the various stages of participatory local level planning, the similar procedure is followed in the health sector starting from identification of felt needs of the community about health to final approval of health project and funds by the DPC.

During 2004-05, local governments together formulated 13267 projects for the health sector with an outlay of 9662 lakhs rupees. Table 7 shows the local government-wise outlay set apart for health during 2004-05 (Government of Kerala, 2005).

Table 7: Local Self-government-wise Outlay on Health during 2004-05, Kerala

Institutions	Projects (Numbers)	2004-05 (Rs. In lakhs)
Grama Panchayat	10865	5524
Block Panchayat	1381	1326
District Panchayat	377	1256
Sub Total	12623	8106
Municipality	594	928
Corporation	50	630
Total	13267	9664

Source: Government of Kerala (2005).

Impact of Decentralized Planning on Health Sector in Kerala

What has been the impact of decentralized planning on the health sector so far? It is difficult to assess the performance of the health sector under decentralized planning in Kerala. There are few scientifically valid studies to assess the performance. The available results thus far have been mixed. The experience shows that local governments have been successful in providing basic minimum infrastructure services like water supply, sanitation, housing and buildings for hospitals and dispensaries. Although there is no visible improvement in the quality of services, access to health services has shown an improvement. The disadvantaged groups like Scheduled Castes (SCs) have not derived much benefit in public service delivery in education and health (Eapen and Thomas, 2005). There seems to be difficulties encountered by the local governments to manage and improve performance of health personnel. Unlike many examples of successful models of decentralization in other sectors such as water supply and sanitation, decentralized planning for health from below has not yet been evolved.

The innovations in health interventions in local governments include introduction of health cards, school health programmes and to a lesser extent health co-operatives. A large majority of the health projects have been limited to improvement of infrastructure and purchase of equipment. In the health sector, Malappuram District Hospital seems to be a unique model as reflected by its success in generating huge revenues from various local governments in the districts and non-resident Indians (NRIs).

Let us look at the empirical evidence of the impact of decentralization of the healthcare sector.

A study undertaken in four districts of Kerala found that decentralization led to greater flow of funds to the local bodies, more autonomy over spending decisions, faster project implementation, less corruption, and greater advocacy of preventive and curative care and provision of family planning services through PHCs. The elected representatives of local government are aware of issues related to decentralization and health such as role of non-governmental health services, user fees, management of user fees etc. However, the study identified the problems of benefits spill over in the case of taluk hospitals and existing inequalities in the distribution of hospitals (Narayana and Kurup, 2000).

Another study found some of the positive effects of decentralized planning on local governments and communities in terms of increased space and enhanced range of choice in overall planning process in general and health in particular. However, intended benefits were not fully realized due to lack of expertise and lack of full involvement by doctors. Since health is a technical subject, the local governments should have expertise to plan at the local levels (Ramankutty, 2002). Another study had a similar finding that suggests that the reasons for low direct investment in health are the lack of technical expertise and lack of involvement by the health personnel (Varghese, 2002).

Varatharajan *et al* (2002) found inadequate allocation of resources to the health sector in general. In addition, there are problems with small-sized health projects with very limited resources per project. The study suggests that there could be an improvement in patient flow as well as reduction in costs with a higher investment in health sector.

In spite of methodological weaknesses, an important study to assess the performance of primary health centers (PHCs) under decentralized government in Kerala is by Varatharajan *et al.* (2004). The impact is analyzed by comparing the performance of PHCs under two contrasting scenarios of good and not-so-good panchayat support. The study has utilized various sources of data–published and unpublished government data, panchayat development reports, panchayat and PHC records, facility check list, and key informant and client exit interviews.

The findings suggest that panchayats in Kerala have allocated a lower proportion of resources to health as compared to the allocation by the state government prior to decentralization. PHCs were funded to the extent of 0.7-2.7 per cent of the total costs. Even the average annual rate of growth of panchayat resources is four times higher than the rate of growth of health resources–31 per cent versus 8 per cent.

The overall conclusion is that decentralization has not brought about any significant change (qualitative or quantitative) to the health sector. Only in few places did active support from panchayats exist with corresponding good performance of PHCs. In most of the cases, panchayat support to PHCs is passive leading to insignificant change in the performance (Varatharajan *et al.* 2004).

A recent study found that decentralization has failed to move power from the centre to community representatives, especially women, and healthcare providers (Nanda, 2005).

Lessons Learnt and Government Action

There are various lessons learnt during the decentralization process, and the government has responded to meet some unexpected challenges by taking new initiatives.

The first issue to be dealt with is the roles and responsibilities of various actors in the health sector and in local governments. So far, there have not been clear-cut rules about the planning and implementation functions of these actors. While the Health Department has been successful in transferring the funds, it has not played a proactive role in facilitating decentralization of the health sector. Similarly, the local governments have been successful in providing and improving the facilities of the hospitals, but they have not been able to successfully manage and supervise the health personnel. This is partly due to the deficiency of expert knowledge of health by the local governments, hierarchy differential between health personnel and local governments (e.g. the Secretary of the local government is junior in status when compared to the medical officer), and no measurable performance standards of personnel. To respond to these challenges, the government has proposed to conduct joint training for elected representatives and health personnel focusing on behavioural aspects and clarifications of roles. In addition, the government has provided a Code of Conduct in Panchayat Raj and the Municipality Acts delineating the roles and responsibilities of local governments and other professionals. The government has also taken initiative in the preparation of a detailed manual for running institutions on the lines of the Election Manual. It is to be noted that much more needs to be done to integrate functioning of different officials and institutions with local governments.

A related issue is the extent of autonomy by the local governments in decision-making. The health department undertakes the hiring and placement of staff. The centralized cadre management of health providers may hinder adequate delivery of minimum level of services to the people (Nayyar, 2001; Kutty, 2001). As a result, the local governments in backward areas face difficulties in filling up the posts of doctors and other health personnel. Similarly, the health department takes decisions on the procurement and distribution of drugs and local governments have no freedom on the choice of drugs. Also, the existing Public Health Acts have not been modified to involve local governments. Moreover, the devolution of power and authority transfers only preventive and promotive healthcare to local governments. Curative services in large number of smaller hospitals at the secondary level, catering mostly to the rural population, still remain with the government (Saxena, 2006).

It is also frustrating to note that the government directly controls all the centrally sponsored schemes for control of communicable diseases and the PRIs have a negligible role. This reflects a failure to integrate state and centrally sponsored schemes, on the one hand, and to integrate these with the local plans in the health sector. As a result there seems to be inadequate efforts in the health sector projects to cater to the needs of maternal and child health (Elamon and Ekbal, 2000). Maternal and child health are vital issues that need serious attention.

Another important issue is the weak monitoring and evaluation of health projects, especially at the community level. The government has involved Kudumbashree programme (women's self-help groups) to improve access to health services. The Kudumabshree programme could be involved in community-based health insurance and monitoring of health. The government has recently approved a community-led monitoring system in public health institutions.

The issue of integration of services within the health sector is a major issue. At the local government level neither there is evidence of integration of various health facilities (allopathic, ayurvedic and homeopathic), nor the integration of various societies of the Central Government such as tuberculosis, AIDS, blindness, leprosy etc. with the local governments.

Since health facilities were not uniform across the state at the time of decentralization, there is a possibility that the disparity in health facilities has widened over time. Specifically, the health centres under local governments with low initial level of health facility are likely to perform poorly as compared to the health centres with better initial level of health facilities under local governments. The former needs higher allocation of funds and pressures to mobilize more resources compared to the latter. To help fill these gaps, the government has taken initiative on evolving a minimum standard of facilities and services at the hospital levels and to publish a Citizen's Charter regarding the provision of these services by the local governments. The local governments have been given power to mobilize resources through collection of local taxes. However, local resource mobilization has been very weak.

Participation is central to the decentralization process. But the quality of participation seems to be declining with people attending grama sabha and ward sabha more in expectation of benefits than with the objective of shaping investment decisions. Social auditing is also weak. Similarly, another important element of decentralization is accountability. Although some systems of accountability are in place (e.g. Local Fund Audit and Performance Audit), they do not seem to be functioning effectively in local governments.

According to the recent Economic Survey of Kerala, the fiscal crisis of the state is getting transmitted to the local governments through fund flow problems and treasury restrictions (Government of Kerala, 2005). The fiscal decentralization scenario is disturbing in Kerala: (a) the percentage of local government expenditure to total government expenditure has declined between 1998-99 and 2002-03, reflecting a decline in expenditure decentralization, and (b) the average rate of growth in the tax revenue of PRIs has been negative during the same period, reflecting unfavourable trend in revenue decentralization (Oommen, 2006). Given this fiscal crisis in Kerala, financial sustainability of local governments is going to be a huge challenge. It is high time to look for innovative models of resource mobilization including community-based health insurance schemes. The PRIs are carrying out a number of activities related to water, roads, street lighting, drainage and solid waste that directly impact the primary health component. Thus, the government could consider delegating power to PRIs to plan, manage and run various welfare programmes including community health insurance, especially for the poor.

Conclusions

There is no doubt that decentralization of the healthcare sector has been very comprehensive in Kerala. Kerala has demonstrated a unique example of progressive empowerment of PRIs.The devolution of administrative, political and financial decision-making power to local governments has taken place only in Kerala. Except medical colleges and a few general hospitals, all health institutions are managed and supervised by local governments. The decentralization process is successful in bringing government closer to the people. It has also created a political structure that is perceived to be transparent and accountable to the disadvantaged people. Decentralization has taken firm roots in Kerala.

Given the lack of data at the local level, it is difficult to evaluate the successes and prospects of decentralization for the provision of health services. The existing evidence suggests that the impact of decentralization on the health sector is mixed. While access to, and outreach of, health services have improved, there had not been any visible improvement in the quality of services. The local governments have been successful in providing basic infrastructure facilities like water supply and sanitation, housing, and buildings for hospitals and dispensaries. However, local governments have been less successful in managing and controlling the health personnel. There are only a few successful interventions in the field of health sector. The pattern of local government spending suggests that health sector is receiving a low priority as compared to other sectors. This clearly indicates that the resource constraints may continue to affect the access and quality of services even in a decentralized system. Moreover, unlike some other sectors, the methodology of planning for health has not yet been developed. Given the fact that such a large-scale decentralization always brings with it conflicts and dilemmas (Kannan, 2000), it is noteworthy that the Government of Kerala has responded to several challenges constantly and carefully.

With reference to Haryana, Rajasthan, Maharashtra and Karnataka, there have been instances where the dominant rural elites continue to dominate the PRIs either through capturing the seats of power or acting as pressure groups. This problem is further compounded by their class and caste status in the rural social structure. The attendance in the meetings of gram sabha was considerably low, especially in case of women (Lele, 2001; Nambiar, 2001; Deshpande and Murthy 2002). In the case of Kerala, however, PRIs were able to perform their roles effectively to address the local needs, and the rural elites did not obstruct the functioning of the PRIs. However, even in Kerala, the participation of women in gram sabhas is relatively low, and decentralization has not succeeded to ensure sufficient participation of women in the planning process (Isaac *et al.* 1999; Chathukulam and John, 2000). This is indeed surprising given the fact that one-third of the seats in local governments are reserved for women and there is provision in local level plans for a special Women Component Plan amounting to 10 per cent of the plan outlay. This opportunity is not being sufficiently tapped by the women's organizations in Kerala. The feminist groups and development NGOs in Kerala should play a supportive and complementary role to the PRIs to facilitate active community participation in health and other development programmes.

In order to continue the momentum of the current institutional phase of strengthening decentralization process in Kerala, the government has to respond strategically and quickly to meet the challenges during the decentralization process. In the health sector, the following issues need to be faced upfront: clear roles and responsibilities of local governments and health personnel at various levels, decentralization of cadre management of health providers (e.g. PRIs autonomy to appoint doctors, specialists and para-medics), PRIs autonomy in the implementation of centrally sponsored schemes for control of communicable diseases, monitoring and evaluation of health sector, mobilization of resources, minimum standards for facilities and services in various levels, innovations in involving Kudumbashree in the provision of health services, measures to reduce inequalities in health facilities, making gram sabhas more effective and responsive by ensuring participation of women and other most deprived sections of the society, and provision of better quality healthcare. Given the current fiscal crisis in Kerala, financial sustainability of local governments is going to be a huge challenge. The PRIs need to mobilize resources for strengthening public health system. Government of India should play an important role in facilitating the decentralization process by providing expertise and financial support.

Most states in India are lagging in transferring substantial powers and autonomy to the local governments as envisaged in the Constitutional amendments of 1992 (UNDP, 2000; Government of India, 2002a & 2005). However, the demands at the grassroot for greater empowerment of panchayats have begun to grow, and marginalized groups and women in panchayats have increasingly begun to exercise power and are becoming important votaries of decentralization (Mathur, 2006). In many states PRIs are successfully monitoring and implementing various health programmes (Gupta and Gumber, 1999). Panchayati Raj Institutions (PRIs) have to be empowered in all the states in India. They need to be involved in the delivery of basic services such as education and health to the poor as well as to build capacity. The PRIs should be involved to implement the centrally-sponsored schemes designed to serve national priorities. Given the vastness and diversity of the country, PRIs are the answer to an effective and efficient delivery of services. The Central Government and state governments should play an activist facilitator role in ensuring institutionalization of decentralized governance. Since accountability and corruption are central issues in the process of decentralization, decentralization at the level of PRIs should be done with a lot of preparation to be effective (Satia, Mavlankar and Bhat, 1999; Mavlankar, 1999). The experience of Kerala demonstrates this important aspect for the successful implementation of projects at the panchayat level.

The decentralization efforts in various states in India can take due advantage of the increased resource commitments to social sector initiatives by the present United Progressive Alliance (UPA) government. The Union Budget 2006-07 has streamlined various initiatives into eight flagship programmes, including the National Rural Health Mission (NRHM) that was launched last year. The flagship programmes should help the government in making substantial savings as well as reducing administrative delays in the implementation phase. The NRHM aims to provide effective healthcare to the entire rural population, with special focus on 18 states having weak public health indicators and/or weak infrastructure. While very little budgetary support was made available to this scheme last year, government spending in this year's budget has increased by 22 per cent of the planned healthcare outlay. This increase in planned outlay in the health and family welfare programmes is predominantly to enhance the primary healthcare services under its flagship programmes.

Following a 'bottom-up' approach to development, the NRHM includes ambitious goals, including decentralization of healthcare, with districts and village health plans, the training of over 250,000 Accredited Social Health Activists (ASHA) at the village/hamlet level, and new Indian Public Health Standards strengthening the capacity of PRIs in governing healthcare (Government of India, 2005a). ASHA is expected to be selected by the PRIs at village-level and be accountable to them. ASHA is also expected to work in coordination with the existing anganwadi workers and Auxiliary Nurse Midwives. ASHA's work is expected to include creating awareness about basic nutrition, sanitation, counselling women on birth preparedness, importance of safe delivery, escorting children and pregnant women requiring treatment, providing primary medical care for minor ailments and collection of information on births and deaths. The increased budgetary support in this year's budget is expected to make ASHA fully functional and to provide round-the-clock services in block level community health centres. Given the fact that most of the states have stagnant health indicators and medical care is now the second most common cause of family debt, it is an opportune moment to take advantage of the implementation of the NRHM by the states and to transfer power and autonomy (political, administrative and fiscal) to the PRIs by the states in accordance with the guidelines of the 73rd Constitutional Amendment. A strong community-controlled accountability mechanism (or community vigilance) is necessary to monitor the activities of PRIs. A conducive policy environment in this respect is the introduction of Right to Information Bill, which is expected to make the functioning of the PRIs more transparent at grassroots level. All these measures will ensure effective spending on healthcare as well as improved health status of the poor and disadvantaged, especially women and children.

REFERENCES

Akin J., Hutchinson P., and Strumpf K., 'Decentralization and Government Provision of Public Goods: The Public Health Sector in Uganda', *Journal of Development Studies*, Vol. 41, No. 8, 2005.

Asthana A.N., 'Decentralization and Supply Efficiency: The Case of Rural Water Supply in Central India', *Journal of Development Studies*, Vol. 39, No. 4, 2003.

Bagchi A, 'Rethinking Federalism: Changing Power Relations between the Centre and the States', *Publius: The Journal of Federalism*, Vol. 33, No. 4, 2003.

Bardhan P., 'Decentralization of Governance and Development', *Journal of Economic Perspectives*, Vol. 16, No. 4, 2002.

Bardhan P. and Mookherjee D., 'Decentralization and Accountability in Infrastructure Delivery in Developing Countries', *Economic Journal*, Vol. 116, No. 598, 2006.

Beall Jo, 'Decentralizing Government and Decentering Gender: Lessons from Local Government Reform in South Africa', *Politics and Society*, Vol. 33, No. 2, 2005.

Bird R. and Vaillancourt F., Fiscal Decentralization in Developing Countries, Cambridge University Press, Cambridge, New York and Melbourne, 1998.

Chathukulam J. and John M.S., 'Empowerment of Women Panchayat Members: Learning from Kerala (India)', *Asian Journal of Women's Studies*, Vol. 6, No. 4, 2000.

Chattopadhyay R. and Duflo E., 'Women as Policy Makers: Evidence from a Randomized Policy Experiment in India', *Econometrica*, Vol. 72, No. 5, 2004.

Crook R. and Manor J., Democracy and Decentralization in South Asia and West Africa: Participation, Accountability and Performance, Cambridge University Press, 1998.

deSouza P.R., 'The Struggle for Local Government: Indian Democracy's New Phase', *Publius: The Journal of Federalism*, Vol. 33, No. 4, 2003.

Deshpande S.V. and Murthy G.B.V., 'Pressure from Below: Decentralized Governance in Karnataka', *Economic and Political Weekly*, May 4, 2002.

Dethier Jean-Jacques(ed), Governance, Decentralization and Reform in China, India and Russia, Kluwer Academic Publishers: Boston, Dordrecht, London, 2000.

Eapen M. and Thomas S., Gender Analysis of Selected of Selected Gram Panchayats Plan-Budgets in Trivandrum District, Kerala, Discussion Paper 11, Human Development Resources Centre, UNDP, New Delhi, 2005.

Elamon J. and Ekbal B., Health Sector Reforms and Local Level Planning: Experience of Kerala, Paper presented at the International Conference on Democratic Decentralization, State Planning Board, Thiruvananthapuram, May 23-27, 2000.

Government of India, National Human Development Report 2001, Planning Commission, New Delhi, 2002a.

Government of India, National Health Policy–2002, Ministry of Health and Family Welfare, New Delhi, 2002b.

Government of India, Mid-Term Appraisal of 10th Five Year Plan (2002-2007), Planning Commission, New Delhi, 2005.

Government of India, National Rural Health Mission (2005-2012) Mission Document, Ministry of Health and Family Welfare, New Delhi, 2005a.

Government of Kerala, Economic Survey 2004, State Planning Board, Thiruvananthapuram, 2005.

Government of Kerala, Human Development Report 2005, Kerala, State Planning Board, Thiruvananthapuraram, 2006.

Guess G.M., 'Comparative Decentralization Lessons from Pakistan, Indonesia, and the Philippines', *Public Administration Review*, Vol. 65, No. 2, 2005.

Gupta D.B. and Gumber A., 'Decentralizations: Some Initiatives in Health Sector', *Economic and Political Weekly*, Vol. 34, No. 6, 1999.

Isaac T.M.T., Seema T.N., Thampy B. and Anthony M., 'Gender and Decentralized Planning: The Experience of People's Campaign', Paper presented in a seminar, Centre for Development Studies, Thiruvanathapuram, July 22, 1999.

Isaac T.M.T., and Franke R.W., Local Democracy and Development: People's Campaign for Decentralized Planning in Kerala, LeftWord Books, New Delhi, 2000.

Jain S.P., 'The Gram Sabha: Gateways to Grassroots Democracy', *Journal of Rural Development,* Vol. 16, 1997.

Johnson C., Deshingar P. and Start D., 'Grounding the State: Devolution and Development in India's Panchayats', *Journal of Development Studies,* Vol. 41, No. 6, 2005.

Kannan K.P., 'People's Planning, Kerala's Dilemma', *Seminar*, 485, January, 2000.

Lele M.K., 'Local Government Conflict of Interests and Issues of Legitimatisation', *Economic and Political Weekly,* December 22, 2001.

Mahal A., Srivastava V., and Saran D., Decentralization and Public Service Delivery in Health and Education Services: Evidence from Rural India in Dethier J. J. (ed), *Governance, Decentralization and Reform in China, India and Russia,* Kluwer Academic Publishers, Boston, Dordrecht, London, 2000.

Mathur K., 'Empowering Local Government: Decentralization and Governance' in Council for Social Development (ed), India: Social Development Report, Oxford University Press, New Delhi, 2006.

Mavalankar D.V., Management Constraints for Operationalization of Reproductive Health Programme Intervention in PHC Systems in India, Indian Institute of Management (Mimeo), Ahmedabad, 1999.

Nambiar M., 'Making the Gram Sabha Work', *Economic and Political Weekly*. August 18, 2001.

Nanda P., 'Moving Towards the 'Centre': Reproductive Health and Rights in Tanzania and Kerala, India', *Development*, Vol. 48, No. 4, 2005.

Narayana D., and Hari Kurup K.K., 'Decentralization of Healthcare Sector in Kerala: Some Issues', Centre for Development Studies Working Paper Number 298, CDS, Thiruvananthapuram, 2000.

Nayyar K.R., 'Politics of Decentralization: Lessons from Kerala' in Qadeer I, Sen K and Nayyar K.R. (eds) *Public Health and the Poverty of Reforms*, 2001.

Oommen M.A., 'Fiscal Decentralization to the Sub-State Level Governments', *Economic and Political Weekly*, March 11, 2006.

Ramankutty V., 'Reforms and Their Relevance: The Kerala Experience', in Qadeer I., Sen K. and Nayyar K.R. (eds) *Public Health and the Poverty of Reforms*, 2001.

Ramankutty V., Health Planning and Decentralization: The Kerala Experience. Unpublished, 2002.

Sadanandan R. and Shiv Kumar N., 'Rogi Kalyan Samitis: A Case Study of Hospital Reforms in Madhya Pradesh', in Chand Vikram K. (ed) *Reinventing Public Service Delivery in India: Selected Case Studies*, Sage Publications, New Delhi, Thousand Oaks and London, 2006.

Satia J., Mavlankar D.V., and Bhat R., 'Progress and Challenges of Health Sector: A Balance Sheet', Working Paper, Indian Institute of Management, Ahmedabad, 1999.

Saxena K.B., Governance and the Health Sector, in Prasad Sujata and Sathyamala C (eds) *Securing Health for All: Dimensions and Challenges*, Institute for Human Development, New Delhi, 2006.

UNDP, Decentralization in India: Constraints and Opportunities, Discussion Paper Series 1, UNDP: Human Development Resource Centre, 2000.

Varatharajan D., Thankappan K.R., and Jayapalan S., 'Assessing the Performance of Primary Health Centres under Decentralized Government in Kerala, India', *Health Policy and Planning*, Vol. 19, No. 1, pp. 41-51, 2004.

Varatharajan D., Sadanandan R., Thankapan K.R., and Mohanan Nair V., 'Idle Capacity in Resource Strapped Government Hospitals in Kerala: Size, Distribution and Determining Factors', Achutha Menon Centre for Health Sciences Studies, SCTIMST, Thiruvananthapuram, 2002.

Varghese J.J., 'Influence of Provincial Guidelines and Assessment of Local Health Needs on Resource Allocation and Programme Implementation of Decentralized Local Self-Governments in Kerala, India', MPH Dissertation, Achutha Menon Centre for Health Sciences Studies, SCTIMST, Thiruvananthapuram, 2002.

Vijayanand S.M., 'Poverty Reduction through Decentralization: Lessons from the Experience of Kerala State in India', Paper presented in the Asia and Pacific Forum on Poverty: Reforming Policies and Institutions of Poverty Reduction, held at the Asian Development Bank, Manila, February 5-9, 2001.

Westergaard, K. and Alam M.M., 'Local Government in Bangladesh: Past Experience and Yet Another Try', *World Development*, Vol. 23, No. 4, 1995.

Index

Dysentery 16, 27, 78, 105